ILLUSTRATED ELEMENTS OF
ESSENTIAL OILS

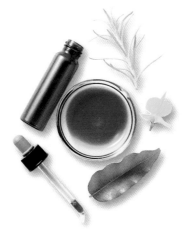

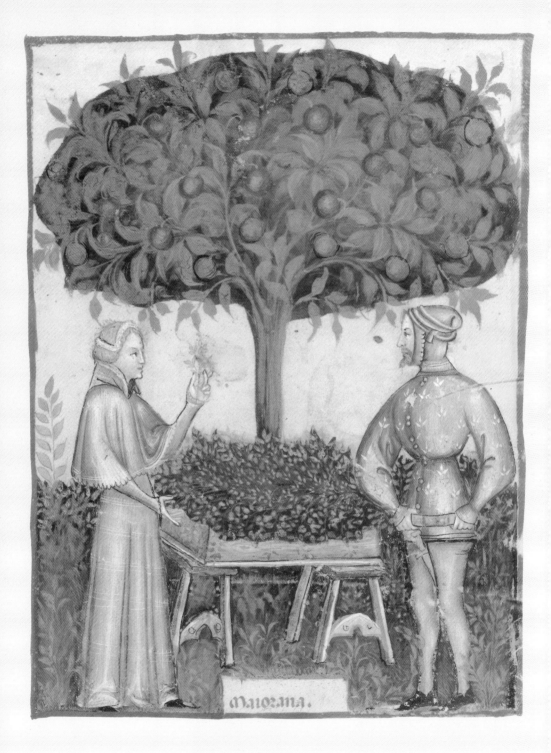

MAIORANA.

ILLUSTRATED ELEMENTS OF
ESSENTIAL OILS

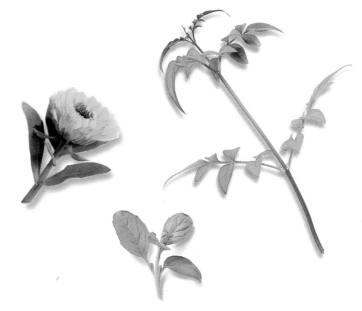

Julia Lawless

ELEMENT

Element
An Imprint of HarperCollins*Publishers*
77–85 Fulham Palace Road
Hammersmith, London W6 8JB

First published in Great Britain in 2002
by Element Books Limited

10 9 8 7 6 5 4 3 2 1

A catalogue record for this book
is available from the British Library

ISBN 0 00 71385 20

Printed and bound in Hong Kong
by Printing Express

Picture credits

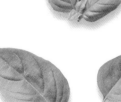

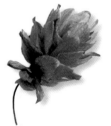

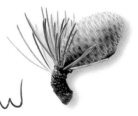

Contents

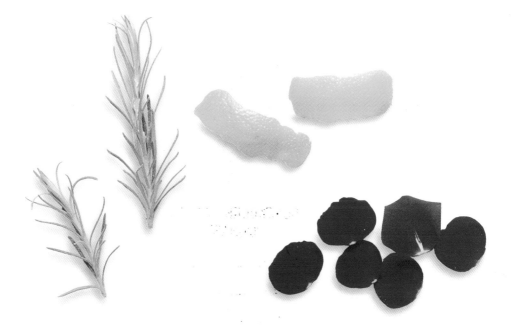

Preface

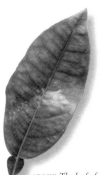

ABOVE *The leaf of the grapefruit tree. Grapefruit oil is a valuable protection against infection.*

Aromatic oils can be found in all the various parts of a plant, including the seeds, bark, root, leaves, flowers, wood, balsam, and resin. The wide range of aromatic materials obtained from natural sources and the art of their extraction and use has developed slowly over the course of time, but its origins reach back to the very heart of the earliest civilizations. The last two decades have seen a growing interest in complementary healing methods and the use of naturally derived products such as essential oils. Aromatherapy, once considered a fringe practice, has become so generally accepted and respected that it is increasingly on offer to hospital patients as part of their treatment. More and more, manufacturers of health products, cosmetics, and perfumes are recognizing the value of essential oils in enhancing the quality and appeal of their products. At the same time, the home use of essential oils has risen dramatically as people discover for themselves the therapeutic benefits and unique esthetic

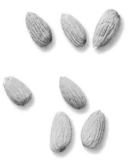

ABOVE *Sweet almond oil is made by pressing almond kernels.*

enjoyment of the oils. Current scientific research into the chemistry and medicinal use of certain essential oils has helped confirm and clarify their precise healing potential. The demand for tea tree oil, for example, has expanded enormously over the last few years as a result of detailed analytical trials – in Australia it has even been hailed as the "antiseptic of the future"! Such studies have highlighted the benefits of essential oils and the need for further research. Cultivation methods, climate, location, precise botanical species, extraction techniques, and handling have all been found to have a profound influence on the final makeup of an oil, thus affecting its fragrance, purity, and therapeutic value.

BELOW *Oil from mandarin leaves is used to strengthen digestive functions.*

How to Use This Book

Essential Oils provides a general introduction to aromatics, showing their changing role throughout history and their modern applications in aromatherapy, herbalism, and perfumery. A therapeutic index lists common complaints, which are grouped according to different parts of the body, with information on how they can be treated using aromatherapy oils. A systematic survey of over 160 essential oils, shown in alphabetical order according to the Latin names of the plants from which they are derived, provides a comprehensive guide, detailing extraction methods, chemistry, and pharmacology.

BELOW As well as discussing the origins and history of aromatherapy, the first part of the book shows you how to use essential oils at home.

Information boxes explain how essential oils work in different parts of the body

BELOW The Therapeutic Index groups ailments according to body systems and lists recommended oils to provide a comprehensive guide to treatment.

Abbreviations indicate the suggested method of application. For key, see page 28

Comprehensive lists of essential oils, grouped by ailment, are an easy-to-follow guide to home use

RIGHT The last part of the book lists 160 essential oils. It indicates how each oil can be used at home, how it was extracted, and with what other oils it is compatible.

This section details the various complaints, listed by body system, that the oil can treat

Special attention should be paid to the Safety Data on each oil

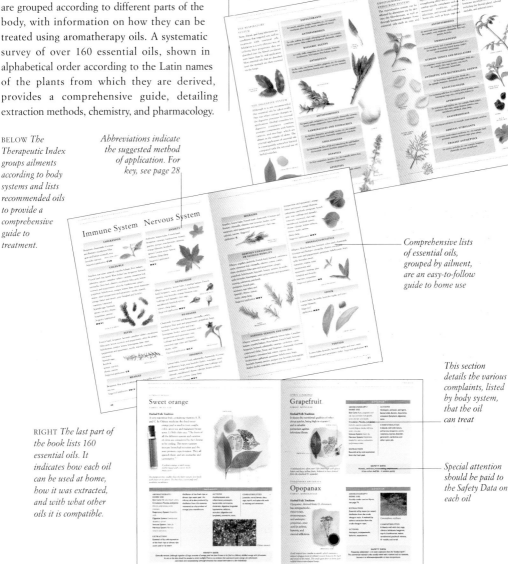

Historical Roots

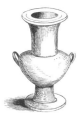

ABOVE *An alabaster vase from ancient Egypt, used to store ointments.*

AROMATIC PLANTS AND OILS *have been used for thousands of years, as incense, perfumes, and cosmetics, and for medical and culinary applications. Natural aromatics and perfume materials were among the earliest trade items of the ancient world, being rare and highly prized. When the Jewish people began their exodus from Egypt to Israel around 1240 BCE, they took many gums and oils with them, together with knowledge of their use. In most early cultures the religious and therapeutic roles of aromatic oils were intertwined. This type of practice is still in evidence: in the East, purifying sprigs of juniper are burned in Tibetan temples; in the West, frankincense is used during the Roman Catholic mass.*

ANCIENT CIVILIZATIONS

The Vedic literature of India, dating from around 2000 BCE, lists over 700 substances including cinnamon, spikenard, ginger, myrrh, cilantro, and sandalwood. But aromatics were considered to be more than just perfumes, and the *Rig Veda* codified their use for both liturgical and therapeutic purposes. The traditional Indian or Ayurvedic system of medicine developed from this understanding of plant lore.

The Chinese also have an ancient herbal tradition that accompanies the practice of acupuncture, the earliest records being in the *Yellow Emperor's Book of Internal Medicine* dating from around 2000 BCE.

But perhaps the most famous and richest associations with the first aromatic materials are found in ancient Egypt. The use of many medicinal herbs is recorded in papyrus manuscripts from the reign of Khufu, around 2800 BCE. Aromatic gums and oils such as cedar and myrrh were used in the embalming process, and the Egyptians were famous for their herbal preparations and ointments.

TREASURES FROM THE EAST

Phoenician merchants brought camphor from China, cinnamon from India, gums from Arabia, and rose from Syria to the civilizations of Greece and Rome. The Greeks learned about perfumery and natural therapeutics from the Egyptians. Herodotus recorded the method of distillation of turpentine in about 425 BCE. Hippocrates, born in Greece in about 460 BCE and revered as the father of medicine, prescribed perfumed fumigations and fomentations.

The Romans were lavish in their use of perfumes, which they used on their hair, bodies, clothes, and beds, and for massage. Roman knowledge of oils spread to Constantinople, where great works were translated into Persian and Arabic and passed on through the Arab world.

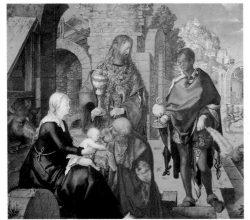

LEFT *In the East, aromatics and perfumes were highly valued commodities used in sacred rites and offered in homage to the gods. This painting by Albrecht Dürer shows the Magi bringing gifts of frankincense and myrrh to the baby Jesus.*

ALCHEMY

The "perfumes of Arabia" spread to Europe at the time of the crusades and became famous throughout Europe. Gradually, the Europeans began to experiment with their own native herbs, such as lavender, sage, and rosemary, which were used for strewing floors and as protection against plague and other infections. Distillation, used to produce pure essential oils and aromatic water, was employed in the practice of alchemy, the hermetic pursuit dedicated to the transformation of base metals into gold, a religious quest in which the stages of distillation were equated with stages of an inner psychic transmutation.

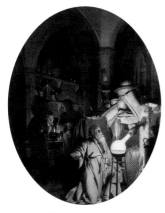

ABOVE *This eighteenth-century painting by Joseph Wright portrays the alchemist's equipment. Retorts and stills were used to extract volatile oils. The stages of distillation were equated with the purified human psyche by alchemists.*

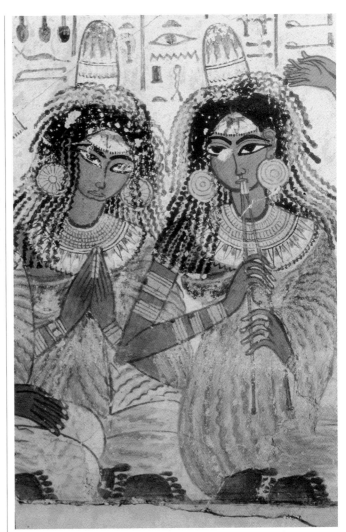

ABOVE *An ancient Egyptian banquet scene, from the fifteenth century BCE, shows women wearing perfume cones on their heads. As the heat melted the cones, their hair and bodies would be waxed and scented.*

THE SCIENTIFIC REVOLUTION

For many centuries, aromatic materials were the main protection against epidemics. The medicinal properties and applications of increasing numbers of new essential oils were analyzed and recorded by the pharmacists. With the scientific revolution of the early nineteenth century, chemists were able to identify the various constituents of the oils and give them specific names. This laid the groundwork for the development of the oils' synthetic counterparts and the growth of the modern drug industry. By the mid twentieth century, essential oils were used only in perfumes, cosmetics, and foodstuffs.

The Birth of Aromatherapy

THE TERM "AROMATHERAPY" *was first coined in 1928 by René-Maurice Gattefossé, a French chemist working in his family's perfumery business. He became fascinated with the therapeutic possibilities of the oils after discovering by accident that lavender was able to heal a severe burn on his hand quite rapidly and help prevent scarring. He also confirmed the discoveries made by Cuthbert Hall in 1904, that many of the essential oils were more effective in their totality than their synthetic substitutes or their isolated active ingredients.*

HERBAL MEDICINE

Aromatherapy is part of the larger field of herbal medicine. The essential oil is only one of many ways in which a plant can be prepared as a remedy. German chamomile, for example, is used extensively as a herbal preparation, as well as being utilized for its volatile oil. It is important to distinguish between an oil's therapeutic qualities and those of the herb taken as a whole. Peppermint oil, for example, is used to treat respiratory conditions as an inhalant, because of its antispasmodic and antiseptic action. But for the longer-term treatment of digestive disorders it is better to use extracts from the whole herb, where the action of the volatile oil is supported by the presence of bitters and tannins.

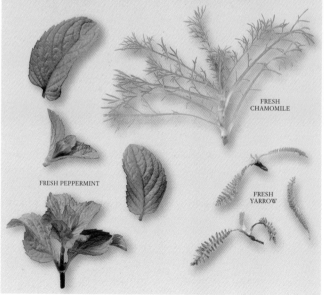

FRESH CHAMOMILE

FRESH PEPPERMINT

FRESH YARROW

In 1964, French doctor and scientist Dr. Jean Valnet used essential oils as part of a program by which he successfully treated specific medical and psychiatric disorders, the results of which were published in the book *Aromatherapie*.

The work of Valnet was studied by Madame Marguerite Maury, who applied his research to her beauty therapy, in which she attempted to revitalize her clients by creating a strictly personal aromatic complex that she tried to adapt to the temperament and particular health problems of each subject.

In many ways "aromatherapy" is a misleading term, suggesting that it is a form of healing that works exclusively through the sense of smell, and on the emotions. In addition to its scent, each essential oil has an individual combination of constituents that interact with the body's chemistry in a direct manner, which then in turn affects certain organs or systems as a whole. For example, when the oils are used externally in the form of a massage treatment, they are easily absorbed through the skin and transported throughout the body. This can be

MADAME MARGUERITE MAURY

Marguerite Maury (1895–1968) was a dedicated and inspired woman who did much to establish the reputation of aromatherapy. She set up the first aromatherapy clinics in France, Britain, and Switzerland and was awarded two international prizes (in 1962 and 1967 respectively) for her studies on essential oils and cosmetology. She focused on the rejuvenating properties of essential oils in her research work, the results of which were published in English as *The Secret of Life and Youth* (1964).

Odor signals are passed *directly* to the limbic system of the brain, evoking an *immediate* emotional or instinctual response.

Aromatic molecules enter the *lungs* and are absorbed via the alveoli into the blood.

The blood is carried to the *heart* and transported throughout the body via the circulatory system.

Different oils have affinities with specific parts of the body – e.g. spices particularly affect the *digestion*.

Waste and toxins are processed by the *liver and kidneys* and eliminated mainly via the lungs, but also in the urine and sweat.

demonstrated by rubbing a clove of garlic on the soles of the feet; the volatile oil content will be taken into the blood and the odor will appear on the breath a little while later.

Essential oils have three distinct modes of action in interrelating with the human body: pharmacological, physiological, and psychological. The pharmacological effect relates to the chemical changes that take place when an essential oil enters the bloodstream and reacts with hormones, enzymes, and so on. The physiological mode is concerned with the way in which an essential oil affects body systems. The psychological effect takes place when an essence is inhaled and an individual responds to its odor.

RIGHT *Airborne aromatic oil molecules interact with the different body systems. Some oils are noted for their particular affinities to specific body systems.*

11

How Essential Oils Work

THE THERAPEUTIC POTENTIAL *of essential oils, like other plant-derived remedies, has yet to be fully realized. Although numerous medical herbs have been utilized since antiquity, many of which have been exploited to provide the biologically active compounds that form the basis of most of our modern drugs, there is still a great deal to be learned about their precise pharmacology. This is particularly true of aromatic oils, which have a concentrated yet multifaceted makeup. Modern research has largely confirmed the traditionally held beliefs regarding the therapeutic uses of particular plants. Like herbal remedies, an essential oil can cover a wide field of activities; the same herb or oil can stimulate certain systems of the body while sedating or relaxing others. In order to gain a clearer understanding of the way essential oils work, and some of their particular areas of activity, it may be helpful to take an overall view of the systems of the human body.*

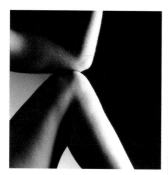

THE SKIN

Skin problems are often the surface manifestation of deeper conditions, such as buildup of toxins in the blood, hormonal imbalance, or nervous and emotional difficulties. Versatile essential oils are able to combat such complaints on a variety of levels. Since essential oils are soluble in oil and alcohol and impart their scent to water, they are an ideal ingredient for cosmetics and skin care as well as for the treatment of specific diseases.

ANTISEPTICS

for cuts, insect bites, blemishes, etc.; for example, thyme, sage, eucalyptus, tea tree, clove, lavender, lemon.

ANTI-INFLAMMATORY

for eczema, infected wounds, bumps, bruises, etc.; for example, German and Roman chamomile, lavender, yarrow.

FUNGICIDAL OILS

for athlete's foot, candida, ringworm, etc.; for example, lavender, tea tree, myrrh, patchouli, sweet marjoram.

GRANULATION STIMULATING OR CICATRIZING (HEALING) AGENTS

for burns, cuts and scars, stretch marks, etc.; for example, lavender, chamomile, rose, orange blossom, frankincense, geranium.

DEODORANTS

for excessive perspiration, cleaning wounds, etc.; for example, bergamot, lavender, thyme, juniper, cypress, Spanish sage, lemongrass.

INSECT REPELLENTS AND PARASITICIDES

for lice, fleas, scabies, ticks, mosquitoes, ants, moths, etc.; for example, spike lavender, garlic, geranium, citronella, eucalyptus, clove, camphor, Atlas cedarwood.

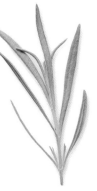

FRESH SPIKE LAVENDER

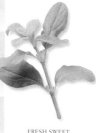

FRESH SWEET MARJORAM

THE CIRCULATION, MUSCLES, AND JOINTS

Essential oils are easily absorbed via the skin and mucosa into the bloodstream, affecting the nature of the circulation as a whole. Oils with a rubefacient or warming effect, such as black pepper, camphor, and sweet marjoram, not only cause better local blood circulation but also influence the inner organs. They bring a warmth and glow to the surface of the skin and can provide considerable pain relief through their analgesic or numbing effect. Such oils can also relieve local inflammation by setting free mediators in the body which in turn cause the blood vessels to expand, so the blood is able to move more quickly and the swelling is reduced. Some oils, such as hyssop, tend to have a balancing or regulating effect on the circulatory system as a whole, reducing the blood pressure if it is too high or stimulating the system if it is sluggish.

HYPOTENSIVES

for high blood pressure, palpitations, stress, etc.;
for example, sweet marjoram, ylang ylang, lavender, lemon.

HYPERTENSIVES

for poor circulation, chilblains, listlessness, etc.; for example,
rosemary, spike lavender, eucalyptus, peppermint, thyme.

RUBEFACIENTS

for rheumatism of the joints, muscular stiffness, sciatica,
lumbago, etc.; for example, black pepper, juniper, rosemary,
camphor, sweet marjoram.

DEPURATIVE OR ANTITOXIC AGENTS

for arthritis, gout, congestion, skin eruptions, etc.;
for example, juniper, lemon, fennel, lovage.

LYMPHATIC STIMULANTS

for cellulitis, obesity, water retention, etc.; for example,
grapefruit, lime, fennel, lemon, mandarin, white birch.

CIRCULATORY TONICS AND ASTRINGENTS

for swellings, inflammations, varicose veins, etc.;
for example, cypress, yarrow, lemon.

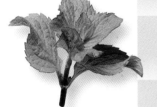

FRESH PEPPERMINT

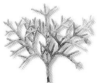

FRESH CYPRESS

FRESH JUNIPER

FRESH LOVAGE

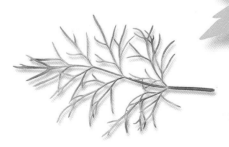

FRESH LEMON

FRESH FENNEL

THE RESPIRATORY SYSTEM

Nose, throat, and lung infections are conditions that respond very well to treatment with essential oils. Inhalation is a very effective way of utilizing their properties; they are absorbed into the blood circulation even faster than by oral application. Most essential oils that are absorbed from the stomach are then excreted via the lungs.

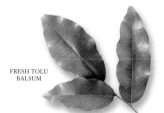

FRESH TOLU BALSUM

THE DIGESTIVE SYSTEM

Although it is not recommended that essential oils be taken orally, they can effect certain changes in the digestive processes by external application. Herbal remedies for digestive complaints combine aromatic components with bitters, tannins, and mucilage, which are absent in the volatile oil alone. The external application of essential oils is consequently somewhat limited compared with the internal use of herbal remedies.

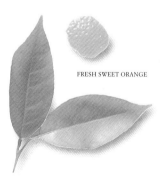

FRESH SWEET ORANGE

EXPECTORANTS

for catarrh, sinusitis, coughs, bronchitis, etc.; for example, eucalyptus, pine, thyme, myrrh, sandalwood, fennel.

ANTISPASMODICS

for colic, asthma, dry cough, whooping cough, etc.; for example, hyssop, cypress, Atlas cedarwood, bergamot, chamomile, cajeput.

BALSAMIC AGENTS

for colds, chills, congestion, etc.; for example, benzoin, frankincense, Tolu balsam, Peru balsam, myrrh.

ANTISEPTICS

for flu, colds, sore throat, tonsillitis, gingivitis, etc.; for example, thyme, sage, eucalyptus, hyssop, pine, cajeput, tea tree, borneol.

FRESH COMMON SAGE

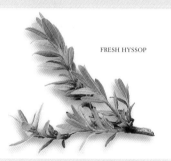

FRESH HYSSOP

ANTISPASMODICS

for spasm, pain, indigestion, etc.; for example, chamomile, caraway, fennel, orange, peppermint, lemon balm, aniseed, cinnamon.

CARMINATIVES AND STOMACHICS

for flatulent dyspepsia, aerophagia, nausea, etc.; for example, angelica, basil, fennel, chamomile, peppermint, mandarin.

CHOLAGOGUES

for increasing the flow of bile and stimulating the gall bladder; for example, caraway, lavender, peppermint, borneol.

HEPATICS

for liver congestions, jaundice, etc.; for example, lemon, lime, rosemary, peppermint.

APERITIFS

for loss of appetite, anorexia, etc.; for example, aniseed, angelica, orange, ginger, garlic.

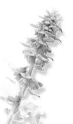

GARLIC

FRESH BASIL

GENITOURINARY/ ENDOCRINE SYSTEMS

The reproductive system can be affected by absorption via the skin into the bloodstream, as well as through hormonal changes. Some essential oils such as rose and jasmine have an affinity for the reproductive system. They have a strengthening effect and also help to combat specific complaints such as menstrual problems, genital infections, and sexual difficulties. Some oils, such as hops, sage and fennel contain plant oils that mimic corresponding human hormones, such as estrogen. Other essential oils are known to influence the levels of hormone secretion of other glands, including the thyroid gland, adrenal medulla, and adrenal cortex.

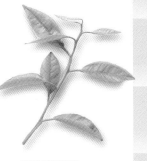

FRESH BERGAMOT

FRESH ROSE PETALS

FENNEL LEAVES AND SEEDS

ANTISPASMODICS

for menstrual cramp (dysmenorrhea), labor pains, etc.; for example, sweet marjoram, chamomile, clary sage, jasmine, lavender.

EMMENAGOGUES

for scanty periods, lack of periods (amenorrhea), etc.; for example, chamomile, fennel, hyssop, juniper, sweet marjoram, peppermint.

UTERINE TONICS AND REGULATORS

for pregnancy, excess menstruation (menorrhagia), PMS, etc.; for example, clary sage, jasmine, rose, myrrh, frankincense, lemon balm.

ANTISEPTIC AND BACTERICIDAL AGENTS

for leucorrhea, vaginal pruritis, thrush, etc.; for example, bergamot, chamomile, myrrh, rose, tea tree.

GALACTAGOGUES

for increasing milk flow; for example, fennel, jasmine, anise, lemongrass (sage, mint, and parsley reduce it).

APHRODISIACS

for impotence and frigidity, etc.; for example, black pepper, cardomon, clary sage, orange blossom, jasmine, rose, sandalwood, patchouli, ylang ylang.

ANAPHRODISIACS

for reducing sexual desire; for example, sweet marjoram, camphor.

ADRENAL STIMULANTS

for anxiety, stress-related conditions, etc.; for example, basil, geranium, rosemary, borneol, sage, pine, savory.

URINARY ANTISEPTICS

for cystitis, urethritis, etc.; for example, bergamot, chamomile, tea tree, sandalwood.

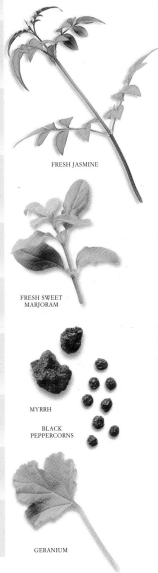

FRESH JASMINE

FRESH SWEET MARJORAM

MYRRH

BLACK PEPPERCORNS

GERANIUM

15

THE IMMUNE SYSTEM

Virtually all essential oils have bactericidal properties, and by promoting the production of white blood cells they can help prevent and treat infectious illness. It is these properties that gave aromatic herbs and oils such high repute with regard to infections such as malaria and typhoid in the tropics and epidemics of plague in the Middle Ages. "People who use essential oils all the time ... mostly have a high level of resistance to illness, catching fewer colds etc., than average and recovering quickly if they do."[1]

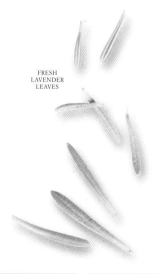

FRESH LAVENDER LEAVES

THE NERVOUS SYSTEM

Research shows that the properties of many oils correspond to the traditionally held views: chamomile, bergamot, and sandalwood were found to have a sedative effect on the central nervous system; jasmine and clove were stimulating. Some oils are known to be "adaptogens," that is, they have a balancing or normalizing effect on the systems of the body. Words like "relaxing" and "uplifting" often relate more to odor description and emotional response than physiological effect, although the two are related.

BACTERIAL AND ANTIVIRAL AGENTS (PROPHYLACTICS)

for protection against colds, flu, etc.; for example, tea tree, cajeput, niaouli, basil, lavender, eucalyptus, bergamot, camphor, clove, rosemary.

FEBRIFUGE AGENTS

for reducing fever and temperature, etc.; for example, angelica, basil, peppermint, thyme, sage, lemon, eucalyptus, tea tree.

SUDORIFICS AND DIAPHORETICS

for promoting sweating, eliminating toxins, etc.; for example, rosemary, thyme, hyssop, chamomile.

SEDATIVES

for nervous tensions, stress, insomnia, etc.; for example, chamomile, bergamot, sandalwood, lavender, sweet marjoram, lemon balm, hops, valerian, lemon.

STIMULANTS

for convalescence, lack of strength, nervous fatigue, etc.; for example, basil, jasmine, peppermint, ylang ylang, orange blossom, angelica, rosemary.

NERVE TONICS

for strengthening the nervous system as a whole; for example, chamomile, clary sage, juniper, lavender, marjoram, rosemary.

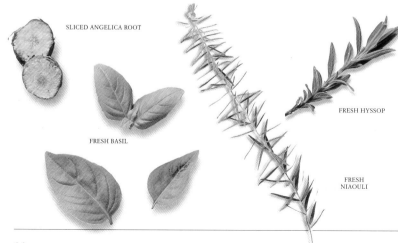

SLICED ANGELICA ROOT

FRESH BASIL

FRESH HYSSOP

FRESH NIAOULI

LEFT *These essential oils have been used to prevent and treat infectious diseases since the Middle Ages. Lavender is also used to strengthen the nervous system as a whole, while basil is known to have a stimulating effect on the central nervous system.*

THE MIND

This is perhaps the most discussed and yet least understood area of activity regarding essential oils. There is no doubt that throughout history aromatic oils have been used for their power to influence the emotions and states of mind: this is the basis for their use as incense for religious and ritualistic purposes.

Recent research in England and Japan has aimed to put traditionally held beliefs into a scientific context. Two types of reactions to odors have been identified: a "hard-wired" response that is instinctual and ingrained from birth, and a "soft-wired" response that is learned or acquired later on.

But to what extent is the effect of a particular oil dependent upon its chemical or physiological make-up, and to what extent does it rely upon a belief or an association? In dealing with the psychological or emotional responses to the scent of a particular oil, it is appropriate to consider the temperament of each individual, rather than predict a set reaction. The effect of an odor on a human being is dependent upon the circumstances in which it is applied, the type of person, his or her mood, and previous associations.

At the Psychology of Perfumery conference 1991, it was generally agreed that "while pharmacological effects may be very similar from one person to another, psychological effects are bound to be different." The effect of an odor on a human being is dependent on a variety of factors, which include:

1 *How the odor was applied.*
2 *How much was applied.*
3 *The circumstances in which it was applied.*
4 *The person to whom it was applied (age, sex, personality type).*
5 *What mood they were in to start with.*
6 *What previous associations they may have with the odor.*
7 *Anosmia, or inability to smell (certain scents).*

When we begin to consider individual needs, essential oils start to demonstrate the versatility of their nature. The rose is a good example of this: a flower associated with beauty, love, and spiritual depth in folklore and religious texts, but also with a long tradition of usage for physical conditions such as skin problems, regulating the female cycle, promoting the circulation, purifying the blood, and as a heart tonic. When we smell the fragrance of the rose, it carries all these rich associations with it, affecting our mind and body simultaneously, as the effect is molded by personal experience.

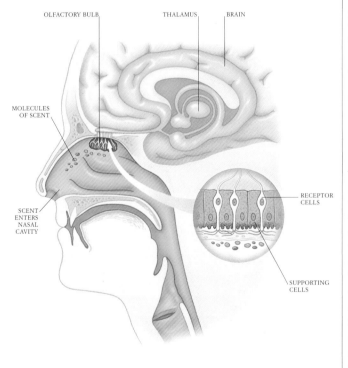

OLFACTORY BULB   THALAMUS   BRAIN

MOLECULES OF SCENT

SCENT ENTERS NASAL CAVITY

RECEPTOR CELLS

SUPPORTING CELLS

ABOVE *Two olfactory nerve tracts run right into the limbic system (the part of the brain concerned with memory and motion), which means that scents can evoke an immediate and powerful response that defies rational analysis.*

How to Use Essential Oils in the Home

ESSENTIAL OILS CAN BE USED at home in a variety of ways. They can be used as perfumes and to revive potpourris; they can be added to the bath and used to make individual beauty preparations. They can also be employed in the treatment of minor first-aid cases and to help prevent and relieve many common complaints such as headaches, colds, period pains, and aching muscles.

MASSAGE

Professional aromatherapists choose specific essential oils to suit the condition and temperament of the patient, which are then blended with a base oil, such as sweet almond oil. The essential oil content in a blend should usually be between 1 per cent and 3 per cent, depending on the type of disorder. Physical ailments such as

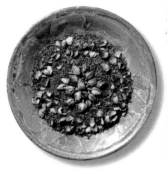

LEFT *A few drops of essential oil added to dried flower petals and seed-heads makes a fragrant pot-pourri.*

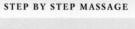

RECIPE

ESSENTIAL OIL	BASE OIL
20 to 60 drops	3½fl oz (100ml)
7 to 25 drops	1fl oz (25ml)
3 to 5 drops	1 tsp (5ml)

STEP BY STEP MASSAGE

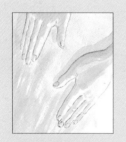

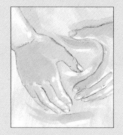

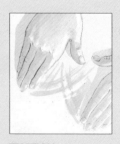

EFFLEURAGE (STROKING MOVEMENTS)
Make sure hands and oil are warm. Use slow, rhythmic strokes to rub the oil well into the skin, keeping the hands in contact with the body.

PETRISSAGE (KNEADING MOVEMENTS)
Suitable for areas of muscular tightness or tension. Use a gentle kneading movement to squeeze and roll the surface skin together with the layers beneath.

FRICTION (CIRCULAR MOVEMENTS)
Especially beneficial for areas of cold, numbness, and poor circulation. Rub the skin in a vigorous circular movement with the flat palms of the hand.

rheumatism demand a stronger concentration than more emotional or nervous conditions. Massage is a relaxing and nourishing experience in itself, and ensures that the oils are effectively absorbed through the skin into the bloodstream.

SKIN OILS AND LOTIONS

The essential oils are prepared much as they would be for a massage, except that the base oil should include the more nourishing oils such as jojoba, avocado, or apricot kernel oil. A gentle circular movement of the fingers is often enough for the oils to be absorbed. Rose and neroli are good for dry or mature complexions; geranium, bergamot, and lemon can help combat acne and greasy skin.

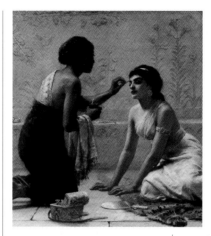

LEFT *Since ancient times, perfumes and cosmetics have been used to enhance appearance.*

HOT AND COLD COMPRESSES

This is an effective way of using essential oils to relieve pain such as backache, rheumatism, earache, and toothache. Fill a bowl with very hot water, then add 4 or 5 drops of essential oil. Dip a folded piece of cloth, absorbent cotton, or a face cloth into the bowl, squeeze out excess water, and place on the affected area.

DIFFERENT SKIN TYPES

OILY SKIN

Oily skin is prone to congestion, often resulting in blemishes and blackheads. Hygiene is very important, but care should be taken not to disturb the natural pH balance of the skin. Astringent and antiseptic essential oils are indicated, such as tea tree bergamot, or geranium. Generally, the base oils should be kept light so that they can be absorbed easily – apricot kernel, peach kernel, or jojoba are ideal.

DRY SKIN

A dry complexion becomes wrinkled more easily than oily skin, especially if it is exposed to too much sun or the effects of central heating. It therefore needs to be moisturized thoroughly and regularly. Dry skin also often tends to be sensitive, so mild essences such as sandalwood, chamomile, and rose are indicated. Rich, nourishing base oils, like hazelnut, avocado, and evening primrose oils, are valuable hydrating agents.

MATURE SKIN

Aging is inevitable, but essential oils can do much to slow down the effects. The regular use of facial treatments containing cytophylactic oils (those that stimulate new cell growth and prevent wrinkles) is vital – such oils include lavender, neroli, and frankincense. Base oils rich in Vitamin E, notably borage and wheatgerm, are especially beneficial for promoting cell regeneration; rosehip seed oil is also indicated.

TRUE LAVENDER

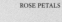

ROSE PETALS

GERANIUM

HAIR CARE

The hair can be enhanced by the use of a few drops of essential oils in the final hair rinse or added straight to a mild shampoo. Oils such as rosemary, West Indian bay, and chamomile all help to condition and encourage healthy hair growth.

RIGHT *An aromatic diffuser with a ribbon wick vaporizes the oil and disperses the scent through the room.*

VAPORIZATION

Scent a room with an oil burner or aromatic diffuser. Alternatively, a few drops of oil can be placed on a light bulb ring or added to a small bowl of water placed on a radiator. Frankincense and cedarwood create a peaceful and relaxed mood.

RECIPE

ALCOHOL-BASED SCALP RUB

This alcohol-based scalp rub can be used to condition the hair or to get rid of unwanted parasites such as lice and fleas. Add 1 tsp (5ml) of essential oil to 3½fl oz (100ml) of vodka.

CONDITIONING TREATMENT

Add about 3 per cent of an essential oil to a base oil such as olive oil with jojoba or sweet almond oil and massage into the scalp, then wrap the head in warm towels for an hour or two.

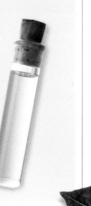

DRIED ROMAN CHAMOMILE

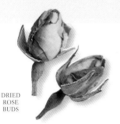

DRIED ROSE BUDS

DOUCHE

In the case of candida or thrush, add between 5 and 10 drops of tea tree to 1¼ pints (1 liter) of warm water and shake well. This mixture can be used on a sitz bath, bidet, or put into an enema/douche pot.

ORANGE BLOSSOM LEAVES

FLOWER WATER

It is possible to make toilet or flower water at home by adding about 20 to 30 drops of essential oil to a 3½ fl oz (100 ml) bottled spring or de-ionized water, leaving it for a few days in the dark and then filtering it using a coffee filter paper. This method can be very helpful in the prevention and treatment of skin conditions such as acne, dermatitis, and eczema, and to tone and cleanse the complexion. Traditional oils include rose, orange blossom, lavender, and petitgrain.

ROSEMARY

LAVENDER

STEAM INHALATION

Especially suited to sinus, throat, and chest infections. Add about 5 drops of an oil such as peppermint or thyme to a bowl of hot water, cover the head and bowl with a towel and breathe deeply for a minute – then repeat. Sitting in a steaming hot bath is another way of inhaling a certain amount of essential oil. Oils such as lemon or tea tree can help to unclog the pores and clear the complexion.

BATHS

Add 5 or 10 drops of oil to the bath-water when the tub is full. Aromatic bathing treats a wide range of complaints, including irritated skin conditions, muscular aches and pains, rheumatism and arthritis.

NEAT APPLICATION

Generally speaking, essential oils are not applied to the skin in an undiluted form. However, lavender, for example, can be applied to burns, cuts, and insect bites. Certain oils, such as jasmine and rose, make excellent perfumes.

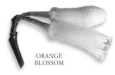

ORANGE
BLOSSOM

CAUTION

Internal use: due to the high concentration of essential oils, it is not recommended that they be taken at home in this manner. Since essential oils are readily absorbed through the skin, they can affect the internal organs by external use.

BELOW *"The Bath" by Alfred George Stevens. Aromatic bathing can relieve stress-related complaints, such as anxiety and insomnia, and aches and pains.*

Creative Blending

ESSENTIAL OILS ARE BLENDED *for two reasons: for their therapeutic effects on a physical condition such as backache; or to create a perfume, which stimulates an emotional or esthetic response. A person who is suffering from a physical complaint also has a psychic or emotional disposition, which will naturally respond in a more subtle way to a particular blend of oils. Similarly, a personal perfume that expresses the unique personality of an individual through fragrance has a generally remedial effect on the person as a whole.*

CORRECT PROPORTIONS

For therapeutic purposes, essential oils are usually diluted before being applied to the skin. To make a massage or body oil, the essential oil or oils should first be mixed with a light base oil such as grapeseed or sweet almond oil. The essential oil content in a blend is usually between 1 and 3 per cent. Physical ailments demand a stronger concentration of essential oils than emotional or nervous conditions.

RIGHT *Correct proportions are important in blending essential oils, as are individual perfume preferences. Some scents can be incompatible – a floral blend, for example, would be unacceptable to most men.*

A SIMPLE BLENDING GUIDE

Each essential oil blends well with members of its own family or group, or with members from a neighboring group, e.g. Citrus and Floral, or Spicy and Woody.

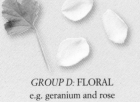

GROUP A: WOODY
e.g. cedarwood and pine

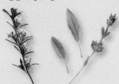

GROUP B: HERBACEOUS
e.g. rosemary and clary sage

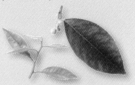

GROUP C: CITRUS
e.g. bergamot and lemon

GROUP D: FLORAL
e.g. geranium and rose

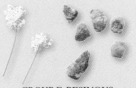

GROUP E: RESINOUS
e.g. galbanum and frankincense

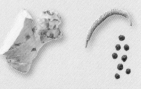

GROUP F: SPICY
e.g. ginger and black pepper

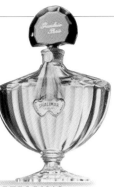

RIGHT *The exotic perfume "Shalimar" by Guerlain is dominated by woody or musky oils. It contains Peru balsam, benzoin, opopanax, vanilla, patchouli, rose, jasmine, orris, vetvier, rosewood, lemon, bergamot, and mandarin.*

SYNERGIES

Some oils blended together have a mutually enhancing effect upon one another. In general, oils of the same botanical family blend well together, as do those that share common constituents, such as the camphoraceous oils. Some oils, such as rose, jasmine, oakmoss, and lavender, enhance just about any blend.

PERSONAL PERFUMES

An individual fragrance needs the correct balance of color or flavors, and also generally has a theme. A perfume should have a focus around which the other fragrances unite. The overall character of a perfume also benefits from unusual or diverse combinations that can give it character.

PIESSE'S LEGACY

In the nineteenth century, a Frenchman named Piesse classified odors according to the notes in a musical scale. The following list provides a general idea of the dominant character of selected oils.

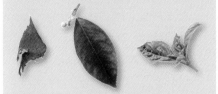

TOP NOTES
A fresh, light, immediate quality
e.g. eucalyptus, lemon, basil

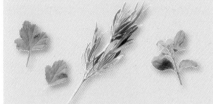

MIDDLE NOTES
The heart of the fragrance
e.g. geranium, lavender, marjoram

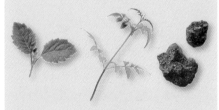

BASE NOTES
A rich, heavy, lingering scent
e.g. patchouli, jasmine, myrrh

A well-balanced perfume is said to contain elements from each of these different categories, the quantities of each determining whether it is a heavy oriental-type scent or a light, floral aroma.

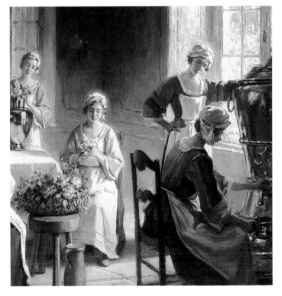

ABOVE *"The Perfume Makers" by Albert Sorkau presents an idealized portrait of the nineteenth-century perfume industry.*

A Guide to Aromatic Materials

OVER THIRTY FAMILIES OF PLANTS, *with about ninety species, represent the main oil-producing group. The majority of spices originate in tropical countries; conversely, the majority of herbs are grown in temperate climates. The same plant grown in a different region and under different conditions can produce essential oils of widely diverse characteristics, which are known as "chemotypes." Common thyme* (Thymus vulgaris), *for example, produces several chemotypes depending on its growth conditions and dominant constituent, notably the citral or linalol types, the thyuanol type, and the thymol or carvacrol type. It is important to know not only the botanical name of the plant from which the oil has been produced, but also its place of origin and main constituents. One of the principal ways of defining the qualities of a particular oil and checking its purity is to ascertain the specific blend of components and to look at its chemical character.*

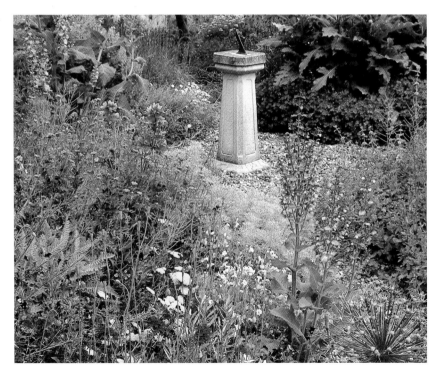

RIGHT *An herb garden with a chamomile path. Most herbs grow in temperate climates, whereas the majority of spices come from tropical climates.*

CHEMISTRY

In general, essential oils consist of chemical compounds that have hydrogen, carbon, and oxygen as their building blocks. These can be subdivided into two groups: the hydrocarbons, which are made up almost exclusively of terpenes (monoterpenes, sesquiterpenes, and diterpenes); and the oxygenated compounds, mainly esters, aldehydes, ketones, alcohols, phenols, and oxides; acids, lactones, sulfur, and nitrogen compounds are sometimes also present.

TERPENES

Common terpene hydrocarbons include limonene (antiviral, found in 90 per cent of citrus oils) and pinene (antiseptic, found in high proportions in pine and turpentine oils); also camphene, cadinene, caryophyllene, cedrene, dipentene, phellandrene, terpinene, sabinene, and myrcene among others. Sesquiterpenes have outstanding anti-inflammatory and bactericidal properties.

GRAPEFRUIT PEEL, LEAF, AND YOUNG FRUIT

ESTERS

Probably the most widespread group found in essential oils, which includes linalyl acetate (found in bergamot, clary sage, and lavender) and geranyl acetate (found in sweet marjoram). They are characteristically fungicidal and sedative, often having a fruity aroma. Other esters include bornyl acetate, eugenyl acetate, and lavendulyl acetate.

ALDEHYDES

Citral, citronellal, and neural are important aldehydes found notably in lemon-scented oils such as melissa, lemongrass, lemon verbena, citronella, etc. Aldehydes in general have a sedative effect; citral has antiseptic properties. Other aldehydes include benzaldehyde, cinnamic aldehyde, cuminic aldehyde, and perillaldehyde.

FRESH PENNYROYAL

KETONES

Some of the most common toxic constituents are ketones, such as thujone found in mugwort, tansy, sage and wormwood; and pulegone found in pennyroyal and buchu. Nontoxic ketones include jasmone (in jasmine) and fenchone (in fennel oil). Other ketones include camphor, carvone, methone, and pinocamphone.

FRESH SPIKE LAVENDER

ALCOHOLS

These compounds have good antiseptic and antiviral properties with an uplifting quality; they are also generally nontoxic. Among the most common terpene alcohols are linalol (in rosewood, linaloe, and lavender), citronellol (in rose, lemon, eucalyptus and geranium) and geraniol (found in palmarosa); also borneol, methol, terpineol, nerol, farnesol, vetiverol, benzyl alcohol, and cedrol.

PHENOLS

These tend to have a bactericidal and strongly stimulating effect, but can be skin irritants. Common phenols include eugenol (found in clove and West Indian bay), thymol (found in thyme), carvacrol (found in oregano and savory); also methyl eugenol, methyl chavicol, anethole, safrole, myristicin, and apiol among others.

FRESH SUMMER SAVORY

OXIDES

By far the most important oxide is cineol (or eucalyptol). It has an expectorant effect, well known as the principal constituent of eucalyptus oil. It is also found in a wide range of other oils, especially those of a camphoraceous nature such as rosemary, bay laurel, tea tree, and cajeput. Other oxides include linalol oxide found in hyssop (decumbent variety), ascaridol, bisabolol oxide, and bisabolone oxide.

FRESH BAY LEAVES

FRESH ROSEMARY

Methods of Extraction

THE TERM "ESSENTIAL OIL" *is loosely applied to all aromatic products or extracts that are derived from natural sources. This is not strictly accurate, since many fragrance products, although they are used by the perfumery industry, are only partially composed of essential oils. The terms "concrete", "absolute", and "resinoid" should be used to denote a type of product that contains a mixture of volatile and nonvolatile components, such as wax or resin, but in the marketplace this is often not the case. Some plant materials, especially flowers, are subject to deterioration and should be processed as soon as possible after harvesting; others, including seeds and roots, are stored or transported for extraction. The extraction method used depends on the quality of the material being used and the type of aromatic product that is required.*

ESSENTIAL OILS

An essential oil is extracted from the plant material by two main methods: by simple expression or pressure, as is the case with most of the citrus oils; or by steam, water, or dry distillation. The majority of oils are produced by distillation. This process isolates only the volatile and water-insoluble parts of the plant – many other constituents are consequently excluded.

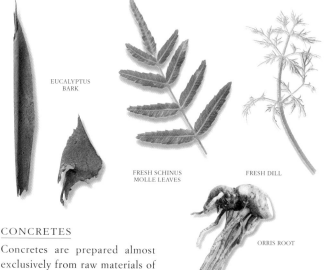

EUCALYPTUS BARK

FRESH SCHINUS MOLLE LEAVES

FRESH DILL

ORRIS ROOT

MARIGOLD FLOWER

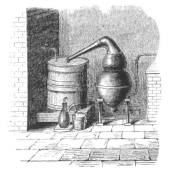

ABOVE *This type of apparatus, with a false bottom, was used for the distillation of plants such as peppermint and lavender.*

CONCRETES

Concretes are prepared almost exclusively from raw materials of vegetable origin, such as the bark, flower, leaf, herb, or root. The aromatic plant material is subjected to extraction by hydrocarbon-type solvents, rather than distillation or expression. This is necessary when the essential oil is adversely affected by hot water and steam, as is the case with jasmine. It also produces a more true-to-nature fragrance.

RESINOIDS

Resinoids are prepared from natural resinous material by extraction with a hydrocarbon solvent, such as petroleum or hexane. Typical resinous materials are balsams (Peru balsam), resins (amber), oleoresins (turpentine), and oleo gum resins (myrrh). They can be viscous liquids, semisolid, or solid, but are usually homogenous masses of noncrystalline character.

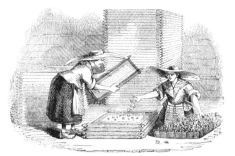

RIGHT *True pomades are the products of a process known as enfleurage, in which a layer of fat is saturated with fragrance from cut flowers. This process is virtually obsolete today.*

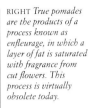

FRESH MASTIC

POMADES

Pomades were made by placing a coating of odorless fat on glass. Freshly cut flowers, laid on the fat, saturated it with their volatile oils. The fat was then treated with alcohol to produce pure absolutes.

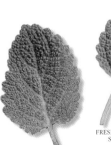

PERU BALSAM
LEAVES

ABSOLUTES

An absolute is obtained from the concrete by a second process of solvent extraction, using pure alcohol in which the unwanted wax is only slightly soluble. A further process of molecular distillation can be used to remove every last trace of nonvolatile matter. The alcohol is recovered by evaporation, which requires a gentle vacuum towards the end of the process.

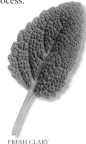

FRESH CLARY
SAGE

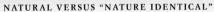

NATURAL VERSUS "NATURE IDENTICAL"

Many perfumes or oils, once obtained from flowers such as gardenia and lilac, are nowadays produced almost entirely synthetically. These chemically constructed "nature identical" products are much cheaper to produce.

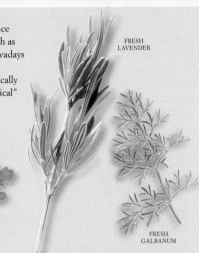

FRESH
LAVENDER

FRESH
GERANIUM

FRESH
GALBANUM

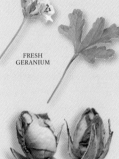

DRIED ROSE
BUDS

Most "nature identical" oils are said to be about 96 per cent pure or accurate, yet it is the remaining 4 per cent, comprising the trace elements, that often defines a fragrance. "Nature identical" oils cannot be used therapeutically.

Therapeutic Index

ESSENTIAL OILS CAN BE USED *to treat a wide range of common complaints, including those listed on the following pages. Special care must be taken regarding the use of oils that can cause irritation in concentration, and oils known to be phototoxic, such as bergamot and lemon. Before using a particular oil, consult the Safety Guidelines. Many of the conditions mentioned in the following pages could benefit from aromatherapy used with other forms of treatment, such as diet, exercise, and herbal medicine.*

ABBREVIATED TERMS USED IN THIS SECTION

B	BATH	**I**	INHALATION *(STEAM)*
C	COMPRESS	**M**	MASSAGE
D	DOUCHE	**N**	NEAT APPLICATION
F	FLOWER WATER	**S**	SKIN OIL/LOTION
H	HAIR CARE	**V**	VAPORIZATION

In the following pages common complaints are grouped according to different parts of the body: Skin Care; Circulation, Muscles, and Joints; Respiratory System; Digestive System; Genitourinary and Endocrine Systems; Immune System; Nervous System. The table above is a guide to abbreviated terms of suggested application, found throughout the Index pages.

THERAPEUTIC GUIDELINES

As a general rule that is in line with the present-day aromatherapy "code of practice", it is best to use essential oils as external remedies only. This is due to the high concentration of the oils and the potential irritation or damage that they can cause to the mucous membranes and delicate stomach lining in undiluted form. There even seems to be some kind of natural order in this scheme, in that volatile oils mix readily with oils and ointments suited to external application, which are absorbed readily through the skin and vaporize easily for inhalation. When inhaled, they can have an effect on the individual's mood or feelings, at the same time causing physiological changes in the body.

These are only superficial guidelines, for there are always exceptions to the rule. Plantain, for example, is an excellent wound-healing herb valuable for external use, although it does not contain any essential oil. Nor can we ignore the fact that a great many aromatic oils are used for flavoring our food and beverages and are consumed daily in minute amounts. For example, peppermint oil is used in a wide variety of alcoholic and non-alcoholic beverages, confectionery, and prepared savory foods, although the highest average use does not exceed 0.104 per cent. Mint oils are used extensively by the pharmaceutical industry in products such as toothpaste, cough and cold remedies, and by the cosmetic industry in soaps, creams, lotions, colognes, and perfumes.

The use of essential oils covers a wide and varied spectrum. On the one hand, they share the holistic qualities of natural plant remedies. On the other hand, they play an active role in the pharmaceutical industry, either in their entirety or in the form of isolated constituents such as "phenol" or "menthol".

It is not the aim of this book to glorify natural remedies (some of which are in fact highly toxic) at the expense of scientific progress, nor to uphold the principles of our drug-oriented culture, but simply to provide information about the multifaceted oils themselves.

CAUTION

Babies and children:
Always increase the dilution for babies and infants to at least half the recommended amount. For babies, avoid the possibly toxic and irritant oils altogether.

SAFETY GUIDELINES

HAZARDOUS OILS
Some oils have high toxicity levels or can cause dermal irritation. Avoid bitter almond, arnica, boldo, broom, buchu, calamus, camphor (brown and yellow), cassia, chervil, cinnamon (bark), costus, deertongue, elecampane, fennel (bitter), horseradish, jaborandi, melilotus, mugwort, mustard, oregano, pennyroyal, pine (dwarf), rue, sage (common), santolina, sassafras, savine, savory, tansy, thuja, thyme (red), tonka, wintergreen, wormseed, and wormwood.

LOVAGE
SPRIG

TOXICITY
The following oils should be used in moderation (only in dilution and for a maximum of two weeks at a time): aniseed, basil (exotic), bay laurel, bay (West Indian), calamintha, camphor (white), cascarilla bark, cassie, cedarwood (Virginian), cinnamon (leaf), clove (bud), cilantro, eucalyptus, fennel (sweet), hops, hyssop, juniper, nutmeg, parsley, pepper (black), sage (Spanish), tagetes, tarragon, thyme (white), tuberose, turmeric, turpentine, valerian.

NEAT APPLICATION
In general, do not apply neat to skin – dilute in carrier oil or cream. Exceptions to this rule include lavender, ylang ylang, and sandalwood. Always do a patch test first, and avoid eyes.

DERMAL/SKIN IRRITATION
Oils that may irritate the skin, especially if used in a high concentration, are: ajowan, allspice, aniseed, basil (sweet), black pepper, borneol, cajeput, caraway, cedarwood (Virginian), cinnamon (leaf), clove (bud), cornmint, eucalyptus, garlic, ginger, lemon, parsley, peppermint, pine needle (Scotch and longleaf), thyme (white), and turmeric. These oils should be used in half the usual recommended dilutions. Always mix them first in a base oil, cream, or gel before applying.

SENSITIZATION
Some oils may cause skin irritation in people with very sensitive skins or can cause an allergic reaction. It is important for those with sensitive skins always to do a patch test before using a new oil to check for individual sensitization. Oils that may cause sensitization: basil (French), bay laurel, benzoin, cade, cananga, cedarwood (Virginian), chamomile (Roman and German), citronella, garlic, geranium, ginger, hops, jasmine, lemon, lemongrass, lemon balm (melissa), litsea cubeba, lovage, mastic, mint, orange, Peru balsam, pine (Scotch and longleaf), styrax, tea tree, thyme (white), Tolu balsam, turmeric, turpentine, valerian, vanilla, verbena, violet, yarrow, and ylang ylang.

CUBEBA
SPRIG

PHOTOTOXICITY
Do not use the following oils either neat or in dilution on the skin, if the area will be exposed to the sun: angelica root, bergamot (not bergapten-free type), cumin, ginger, lemon, lime, lovage, mandarin, orange, and verbena.

PREGNANCY
During pregnancy, use essential oils in half the usual amount. Avoid the following: ajowan, angelica, anise star, aniseed, basil, bay laurel, calamintha, cedarwood (all types), celery seed, cinnamon leaf, citronella, clary sage, clove, cumin, fennel (sweet), hyssop, juniper, labdanum, lovage, marjoram, myrrh, nutmeg, parsley, snakeroot, Spanish sage, tarragon, and thyme (white). Avoid peppermint, rose, and rosemary in the first four months.

HIGH BLOOD PRESSURE
Avoid the following in cases of high blood pressure (hypertension): hyssop, rosemary, sage (Spanish/common), thyme.

EPILEPSY
Avoid the following in cases of epilepsy: fennel (sweet), hyssop, rosemary, and sage (all types).

DIABETICS
Avoid angelica in cases of diabetes.

HOMEOPATHY
Homeopathy is not compatible with black pepper, camphor, eucalyptus, and peppermint.

Skin Care

ACNE

Bergamot, camphor (white), cananga, cedarwood (Atlas, Texas, and Virginian), chamomile (German and Roman), clove bud, galbanum, geranium, grapefruit, helichrysum, juniper, lavandin, lavender (spike and true), lemon, lemongrass, lime, linaloe, litsea cubeba, mandarin, mint (peppermint and spearmint), myrtle, niaouli, palmarosa, patchouli, petitgrain, rosemary, rosewood, sage (clary and Spanish), sandalwood, tea tree, thyme, vetiver, violet, yarrow, ylang ylang.
Suggested application: **M S F B I N**

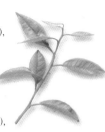

FRESH BERGAMOT

ALLERGIES

Lemon balm, chamomile (German and Roman), helichrysum, true lavender, spikenard.
Suggested application: **M S F B I**

ATHLETE'S FOOT

Clove bud, eucalyptus, lavender (spike and true), lemon, lemongrass, myrrh, patchouli, tea tree.
Suggested application: **S**

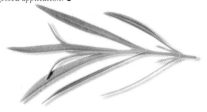

FRESH SPIKE LAVENDER

BALDNESS AND HAIR CARE

West Indian bay, white birch, cedarwood (Atlas, Texas and Virginian), chamomile (German and Roman), grapefruit, juniper, patchouli, rosemary, sage (clary and Spanish), yarrow, ylang ylang.
Suggested application: **S H**

BOILS, ABSCESSES, AND BLISTERS

Bergamot, chamomile (German and Roman), eucalyptus blue gum, galbanum, helichrysum, lavandin, lavender (spike and true), lemon, mastic, niaouli, clary sage, tea tree, thyme, turpentine.
Suggested application: **S C B**

BRUISES

Arnica (cream), borneol, clove bud, fennel, geranium, hyssop, sweet marjoram, lavender, thyme.
Suggested application: **S C**

FRESH LEMON

BURNS

Canadian balsam, chamomile (German and Roman), clove bud, eucalyptus blue gum, geranium, helichrysum, lavandin, lavender (spike and true), marigold, niaouli, tea tree, yarrow.
Suggested application: **C N**

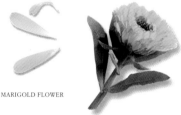

MARIGOLD FLOWER

CHAPPED AND CRACKED SKIN

Peru balsam, Tolu balsam, benzoin, myrrh, patchouli, sandalwood.
Suggested application: **S F B**

CHILBLAINS

Chamomile (German and Roman), lemon, lime, sweet marjoram, black pepper.
Suggested application: **S N**

LEAVES AND FRUIT PEEL OF LIME

COLD SORES/HERPES

Bergamot, eucalyptus blue gum, lemon, tea tree.
Suggested application: **S**

CONGESTED AND DULL SKIN

Angelica, white birch, sweet fennel, geranium, grapefruit, lavandin, lavender (spike and true), lemon, lime, mandarin, mint (peppermint and spearmint), myrtle, niaouli, orange (bitter and sweet), palmarosa, rose (cabbage and damask), rosemary, rosewood, ylang ylang.
Suggested application: **M S F B I**

ROSE PETALS

CUTS/SORES

Canadian balsam, benzoin, borneol, cabreuva, cade, chamomile (German and Roman), clove bud, elemi, eucalyptus (blue gum, lemon, and peppermint), galbanum, geranium, helichrysum, hyssop, lavandin, lavender (spike and true), lemon, lime, linaloe, marigold, mastic, myrrh, niaouli, Scotch pine, Spanish sage,
Levant styrax,
thyme, turpent
vetiver, yarrow.
*Suggested
application:*
S C

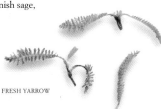

FRESH YARROW

DANDRUFF

West Indian bay, cade, cedarwood (Atlas, Texas, and Virginian), eucalyptus, spike lavender,
lemon, patchouli, rosemary, sage
(clary and Spanish), tea tree.
*Suggested
application:*
S H

FRESH CADE

DERMATITIS

White birch, cade, cananga, carrot seed, cedarwood (Atlas, Texas, and Virginian), chamomile (German and Roman), geranium, helichrysum, hops, hyssop, juniper, true lavender, linaloe, litsea cubeba, mint (peppermint and spearmint), palmarosa, patchouli, rosemary, sage (clary and Spanish), thyme. *Suggested application:* **M S C F B**

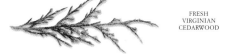

FRESH
VIRGINIAN
CEDARWOOD

DRY AND SENSITIVE SKIN

Peru balsam, Tolu balsam, cassie, chamomile (German and Roman), frankincense, jasmine, lavandin, lavender (spike and true), rosewood, sandalwood, violet.
Suggested application: **M S F B**

ECZEMA

Lemon balm, Peru balsam, Tolu balsam, bergamot, white birch, cade, carrot seed, cedarwood (Atlas, Texas, and Virginian), chamomile (German and Roman), geranium, helichrysum, hyssop,
juniper, lavandin, lavender

FRESH VIOLET

(spike and true), marigold,
myrrh, patchouli, rose
(cabbage and damask),
rosemary, Spanish sage,
thyme, violet, yarrow.
Suggested application: **M S F B**

FRESH
PATCHOULI

EXCESSIVE PERSPIRATION

Citronella, cypress, lemongrass, litsea cubeba, petitgrain, Scotch pine, Spanish sage.
Suggested application: **S B**

FRESH
CYPRESS

GREASY OR OILY SKIN/SCALP

West Indian bay, bergamot, cajeput, camphor (white), cananga, carrot seed, citronella, cypress, sweet fennel, geranium, jasmine, juniper, lavender, lemon, lemongrass, litsea cubeba, mandarin, marigold, mimosa, myrtle, niaouli, palmarosa, patchouli, petitgrain, rosemary, rosewood, sandalwood, clary sage, tea tree, thyme, vetiver, ylang ylang.

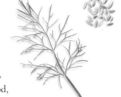

FRESH FENNEL

Suggested application: **M S H F B**

HEMORRHOIDS/PILES

Canadian balsam, copaiba balsam, cilantro, cubeb, cypress, geranium, juniper, myrrh, myrtle, parsley, yarrow.
Suggested application: **S C B**

INSECT BITES

Lemon balm, French basil, bergamot, cajeput, cananga, chamomile (German and Roman), cinnamon leaf, blue gum eucalyptus, lavandin, lavender (spike and true), lemon, marigold, niaouli, tea tree, thyme, ylang ylang.

FRESH CINNAMON

Suggested application: **S N**

INSECT REPELLENT

Lemon balm, French basil, bergamot, borneol, camphor (white), Virginian cedarwood, citronella, clove bud, cypress, eucalyptus (blue gum and lemon-scented), geranium, lavender, lemongrass, litsea cubeba, mastic, patchouli, rosemary, turpentine.
Suggested application: **S V**

FRESH MASTIC

IRRITATED AND INFLAMED SKIN

Angelica, benzoin, camphor (white), Atlas cedarwood, chamomile (German and Roman), elemi, helichrysum, hyssop, jasmine, lavandin, true lavender, marigold, myrrh, patchouli, rose (cabbage and damask), clary sage, spikenard, tea tree, yarrow.

DRIED ROSE BUDS

Suggested application: **S C F B**

LICE

Cinnamon leaf, blue gum eucalyptus, galbanum, geranium, lavandin, spike lavender, parsley, Scotch pine, rosemary, thyme, turpentine.

FRESH COMMON THYME

Suggested application: **S H**

AND GUM INFECTIONS MOUTH/ULCERS

Bergamot, cinnamon leaf, cypress, sweet fennel, lemon, mastic, myrrh, orange (bitter and sweet), sage (clary and Spanish), thyme.
Suggested application: **S C**

PSORIASIS

Angelica, bergamot, white birch, carrot seed, chamomile (German and Roman), true lavender.
Suggested application: **M S F B**

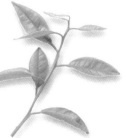

FRESH BERGAMOT

RASHES

Peru balsam, Tolu balsam, carrot seed, chamomile (German and Roman), hops, true lavender, marigold, sandalwood, spikenard, tea tree, yarrow. *Suggested application:* **M S C F B**

RINGWORM

Geranium, spike lavender, mastic, mint (peppermint and spearmint), myrrh, Levant styrax, tea tree, turpentine.

Suggested application: **S H**

FRESH SPEARMINT

SCABIES

Tolu balsam, bergamot, cinnamon leaf, lavandin, lavender (spike and true), lemongrass, mastic, mint (peppermint and spearmint), Scotch pine, rosemary, Levant styrax, thyme, turpentine.

Suggested application: **S**

TRUE LAVENDER
LEAVES

SCARS AND STRETCH MARKS

Cabreuva, elemi, frankincense, galbanum, true lavender, mandarin, orange blossom, palmarosa, patchouli, rosewood, sandalwood, spikenard, violet, yarrow.

Suggested application: **M S**

SLACK TISSUE

Geranium, grapefruit, juniper, lemongrass, lime, mandarin, sweet marjoram, orange blossom, black pepper, petitgrain, rosemary, yarrow.

Suggested application: **M S B**

SPOTS AND BLEMISHES

Bergamot, cade, cajeput, camphor (white), lemon-eucalyptus, helichrysum, lavandin, lavender (spike and true), lemon, lime, litsea cubeba, mandarin, niaouli, tea tree.

Suggested application:

S N

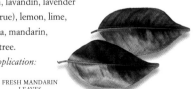

FRESH MANDARIN
LEAVES

TICKS

Sweet marjoram.

Suggested application: **S N**

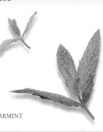

SWEET MARJORAM

TOOTHACHE AND TEETHING PAIN

Chamomile (German and Roman), clove bud, mastic, mint (peppermint and spearmint), myrrh.

Suggested application: **S C N**

VARICOSE VEINS

Cypress, lemon, lime, orange blossom, yarrow.

Suggested application: **S C**

VERRUCAE
(PLANTAR WARTS)

Tagetes, tea tree.

Suggested application: **S N**

LEAVES AND PEEL OF LIME

WARTS AND CORNS

Cinnamon leaf, lemon, lime, tagetes, tea tree.

Suggested application: **S N**

WOUNDS

Canadian balsam, Peru balsam, Tolu balsam, bergamot, cabreuva, chamomile (German and Roman), clove bud, cypress, elemi, eucalyptus (blue gum and lemon-scented), frankincense, galbanum, geranium, helichrysum, hyssop, juniper, lavandin, lavender (spike and true), linaloe, marigold, mastic, myrrh, niaouli, patchouli, rosewood, Levant styrax, tea tree, turpentine, vetiver, yarrow.

Suggested application: **S C B**

WRINKLES AND MATURE SKIN

Carrot seed, elemi, sweet fennel, frankincense, galbanum, geranium, jasmine, labdanum, true lavender, mandarin, mimosa, myrrh, orange blossom, palmarosa, patchouli, rose (cabbage and damask), rosewood, clary sage, sandalwood, spikenard, ylang ylang.

Suggested application: **M S F B**

Circulation, Muscles, and Joints

ACCUMULATION OF TOXINS

Angelica, white birch, carrot seed, celery seed, cilantro, cumin, sweet fennel, grapefruit, juniper, lovage, parsley.
Suggested application: **M S B**

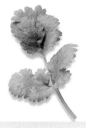

FRESH CILANTRO

ACHES AND PAINS

Ambrette, star anise, aniseed, French basil, West Indian bay, cajeput, calamintha, camphor (white), chamomile (German and Roman), cilantro, eucalyptus (blue gum and peppermint), silver fir, galbanum, ginger, helichrysum, lavandin, lavender (spike and true), lemongrass, sweet marjoram, mastic, mint (peppermint and spearmint), niaouli, nutmeg, black pepper, pine (longleaf and Scotch), rosemary, sage (clary and Spanish), hemlock spruce, thyme, turmeric, turpentine, vetiver.
Suggested application: **M C B**

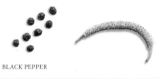

BLACK PEPPER

ARTHRITIS

Allspice, angelica, benzoin, white birch, cajeput, camphor (white), carrot seed, cedarwood (Atlas, Texas, and Virginian), celery seed, chamomile (German and Roman), clove buds, cilantro, eucalyptus (blue gum and peppermint), silver fir, ginger, guaiacwood, juniper, lemon, sweet marjoram, mastic, myrrh, nutmeg, parsley, black pepper, pine (longleaf and Scotch), rosemary, Spanish sage, thyme, turmeric, turpentine, vetiver, yarrow.
Suggested application: **M S C B**

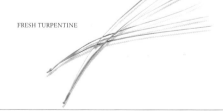

FRESH TURPENTINE

CELLULITIS

White birch, cypress, sweet fennel, geranium, grapefruit, juniper, lemon, parsley, rosemary, thyme.
Suggested application: **M S B**

FRESH JUNIPER

DEBILITY/POOR MUSCLE TONE

Allspice, ambrette, borneol, ginger, grapefruit, sweet marjoram, black pepper, pine (longleaf and Scotch), rosemary, Spanish sage.
Suggested application: **M S B**

AMBRETTE SEEDS

EDEMA AND WATER RETENTION

Angelica, white birch, carrot seed, cypress, sweet fennel, geranium, grapefruit, juniper, lovage, mandarin, orange (bitter and sweet), rosemary, Spanish sage.
Suggested application: **M B**

GOUT

Angelica, French basil, benzoin, carrot seed, celery seed, cilantro, guaiacwood, juniper, lovage, mastic, pine (longleaf and Scotch), rosemary, thyme, turpentine.
Suggested application: **M S B**

FRESH LOVAGE

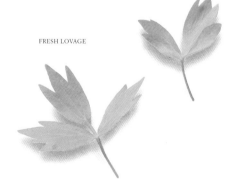

HIGH BLOOD PRESSURE AND HYPERTENSION

Lemon balm, cananga, garlic, true lavender, lemon, sweet marjoram, clary sage, yarrow, ylang ylang.
Suggested application: **M B V**

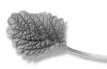

FRESH LEMON BALM

MUSCULAR CRAMP AND STIFFNESS

Allspice, ambrette, cilantro, cypress, grapefruit, jasmine, lavandin, lavender (spike and true), sweet marjoram, black pepper, pine (longleaf and Scotch), rosemary, thyme, vetiver.
Suggested application:
M C B

FRESH JASMINE

OBESITY

White birch, sweet fennel, juniper, lemon, mandarin, orange (bitter and sweet).
Suggested application:
M B

LEAVES AND PEEL OF SWEET ORANGE

PALPITATIONS

Orange (bitter and sweet), orange blossom, rose (cabbage and damask), ylang ylang.
Suggested application: **M**

DRIED ROSE BUDS AND PETALS

POOR CIRCULATION AND LOW BLOOD PRESSURE

Ambrette, Peru balsam, West Indian bay, benzoin, white birch, borneol, cinnamon leaf, cilantro, cumin, cypress, blue gum eucalyptus, galbanum, geranium, ginger, lemon, lemongrass, lovage, niaouli, nutmeg, orange blossom, black pepper, pine (longleaf and Scotch), rose (cabbage and damask), rosemary, Spanish sage, hemlock spruce, thyme, violet.
Suggested application: **M B**

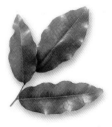

FRESH HEMLOCK SPRUCE

RHEUMATISM

Allspice, angelica, star anise, aniseed, Peru balsam, French basil, West Indian bay, benzoin, white birch, borneol, cajeput, calamintha, camphor (white), carrot seed, cedarwood (Atlas, Texas, and Virginian), celery seed, chamomile (German and Roman), cinnamon leaf, clove bud, cilantro, cypress, eucalyptus (blue gum and peppermint), sweet fennel, silver fir, galbanum, ginger, helichrysum, juniper, lavandin, lavender (spike and true), lemon, lovage, sweet marjoram, mastic, niaouli, nutmeg, parsley, black pepper, pine (longleaf and Scotch), rosemary, Spanish sage, hemlock spruce, thyme, turmeric, turpentine, vetiver, violet, yarrow. *Suggested application:* **M C B**

FRESH PERU BALSAM

SPRAINS AND STRAINS

West Indian bay, borneol, camphor (white), chamomile (German and Roman), clove bud, eucalyptus (blue gum and peppermint), ginger, helichrysum, jasmine, lavandin, lavender (spike and true), sweet marjoram, black pepper, pine (longleaf and Scotch), rosemary, thyme, turmeric, vetiver. *Suggested application:* **C**

35

Respiratory System

ASTHMA

Asafetida, lemon balm, Canadian balsam, Peru balsam, benzoin, cajeput, clove bud, costus, cypress, elecampane, eucalyptus (blue gum, lemon-scented, and peppermint), frankincense, galbanum, helichrysum, hops, hyssop, lavandin, lavender (spike and true), lemon, lime, sweet marjoram, mint (peppermint and spearmint), myrrh, myrtle, niaouli, pine (longleaf and Scotch), rose (cabbage and damask), rosemary, sage (clary and Spanish), hemlock spruce, tea tree, thyme.

Suggested application: **M V I**

SWEET MARJORAM

BRONCHITIS

Angelica, star anise, aniseed, asafetida, lemon balm, Canadian balsam, copaiba balsam, Peru balsam, Tolu balsam, French basil, benzoin, borneol, cajeput, camphor (white), caraway, cascarilla bark, cedarwood (Atlas, Texas, and Virginian), clove bud, costus, cubeb, cypress, elecampane, elemi, eucalyptus (blue gum and peppermint),silver fir, frankincense, galbanum, helichrysum, hyssop, labdanum, lavandin, lavender(spike and true), lemon, sweet marjoram, mastic, mint (peppermint and spearmint), myrrh, myrtle, niaouli, orange (bitter and sweet), pine (longleaf and Scotch), rosemary, sandalwood, hemlock spruce, Levant styrax, tea tree, thyme, turpentine, violet.

Suggested application: **M V I**

DRIED STAR ANISE

CATARRH

Canadian balsam, Tolu balsam, cajeput, cedarwood (Atlas, Texas, and Virginian), cubeb, elecampane, elemi, eucalyptus (blue gum and peppermint), frankincense, galbanum, ginger, hyssop, jasmine, lavandin, lavender (spike and true), lemon, lime, mastic, mint (peppermint and spearmint), myrrh, myrtle, niaouli, black pepper, pine (longleaf and Scotch), sandalwood, Levant sytrax, tea tree, thyme, turpentine, violet.

Suggested application: **M V I**

FRESH ELECAMPANE

CHILL

Copaiba balsam, benzoin, cabreuva, calamintha, camphor (white), cinnamon leaf, ginger, grapefruit, orange (bitter and sweet), black pepper.

Suggested application: **M B**

FRESH CALAMINTHA

CHRONIC COUGHS

Lemon balm, Canadian balsam, costus, cubeb, cypress, elecampane, elemi, frankincense, galbanum, helichrysum, hops, hyssop, jasmine, mint (peppermint and spearmint), myrrh, myrtle, sandalwood, Levant styrax.

Suggested application:

M V I

FRESH GALBANUM FLOWERS

COUGHS

Angelica, star anise, aniseed, copaiba balsam, Peru balsam, Tolu balsam, French basil, benzoin, borneol, cabreuva, cajeput, camphor (white), caraway, cascarilla bark, Atlas cedarwood, eucalyptus (blue gum and peppermint), silver fir, ginger, hyssop, labdanum, sweet marjoram, myrrh, niaouli, black pepper, pine (longleaf and Scotch), rose (cabbage and damask), rosemary, sage (clary and Spanish), hemlock spruce, tea tree.

Suggested application: **M V I**

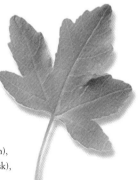

LEVANT STYRAX

CROUP

Tolu balsam.
Suggested application: **M I**

EARACHE

French basil,
chamomile
(German and
Roman), lavender
(spike and true).
*Suggested
application:* **C**

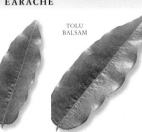

TOLU
BALSAM

HALITOSIS/OFFENSIVE BREATH

Bergamot, cardomon, sweet fennel, lavandin, lavender (spike
and true), mint (peppermint and spearmint), myrrh.
Suggested application: **S**

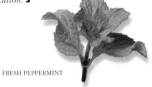

FRESH PEPPERMINT

LARYNGITIS/HOARSENESS

Tolu balsam, benzoin, caraway, cubeb, lemon-scented
eucalyptus, frankincense, jasmine, lavandin, lavender
(spike and true), myrrh, sage (clary and Spanish),
sandalwood, thyme.
*Suggested
application:* **I**

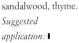

FRESH SPANISH SAGE

SINUSITIS

French basil, cajeput, cubeb, blue
gum eucalyptus, silver fir, ginger,
labdanum, peppermint, niaouli,
pine (longleaf and Scotch), tea tree.
Suggested application: **I**

ROOT OF GINGER

SORE THROAT AND THROAT INFECTIONS

Canadian balsam, bergamot, cajeput, eucalyptus (blue gum,
lemon-scented and peppermint), geranium, ginger, hyssop,
lavandin, lavender (spike and true), myrrh, myrtle, niaouli,
pine (longleaf and Scotch), sage (clary and Spanish),
sandalwood, tea tree, thyme, violet.
Suggested application: **V I**

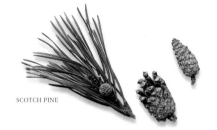

SCOTCH PINE

TONSILLITIS

Bay laurel, bergamot, geranium, hyssop, myrtle, sage (clary
and Spanish), thyme. *Suggested application:* **I**

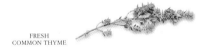

FRESH
COMMON THYME

WHOOPING COUGH

Asafetida, helichrysum, hyssop, true lavender, mastic, niaouli,
rosemary, sage (clary and Spanish), tea tree, turpentine.
Suggested application: **M I**

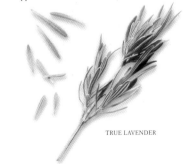

TRUE LAVENDER

Digestive System

COLIC

Star anise, aniseed, lemon balm, calamintha, caraway, cardomon, carrot seed, chamomile (German and Roman), clove bud, cilantro, cumin, dill, sweet fennel, ginger, hyssop, lavandin, lavender (spike and true), sweet marjoram, mint (peppermint and spearmint), orange blossom, parsley, black pepper, rosemary, clary sage.

SPIKE LAVENDER

Suggested application: **M**

CONSTIPATION AND SLUGGISH DIGESTION

Cinnamon leaf, cubeb, sweet fennel, lovage, sweet marjoram, nutmeg, orange (bitter and sweet), palmarosa, black pepper, tarragon, turmeric, yarrow.

Suggested application: **M B**

FRESH TARRAGON

CRAMP/GASTRIC SPASM

Allspice, star anise, aniseed, caraway, cardomon, cinnamon leaf, cilantro, costus, cumin, galbanum, ginger, lavandin, lavender (spike and true), lovage, mint (peppermint and spearmint), orange blossom, black pepper, clary sage, tarragon, lemon verbena, yarrow.*Suggested application:* **M C**

FRESH YARROW

GRIPING PAINS

Cardomon, dill, sweet fennel, parsley.
Suggested application: **M**

HEARTBURN

Cardomon, black pepper. *Suggested application:* **M**

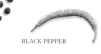

BLACK PEPPER

INDIGESTION/FLATULENCE

Allspice, angelica, star anise, aniseed, lemon balm, French basil, bay laurel, calamintha, caraway, cardomon, carrot seed, cascarilla bark, celery seed, chamomile (German and Roman), cinnamon leaf, clove bud, cilantro, costus, cubeb, cumin, dill, sweet fennel, galbanum, ginger, hops, hyssop, lavandin, lavender (spike and true), lemongrass, linden, litsea cubeba, lovage, mandarin, sweet marjoram, mint (peppermint and spearmint), myrrh, nutmeg, orange (bitter and sweet), orange blossom, parsley, black pepper, petitgrain, rosemary, clary sage, tarragon, thyme, valerian, lemon verbena, yarrow.

FRESH LITSEA CUBEBA

Suggested application: **M**

LIVER CONGESTION

Carrot seed, celery seed, helichrysum, linden, rose (cabbage and damask), rosemary, Spanish sage, turmeric, lemon verbena.

FRESH LEMON VERBENA

Suggested application: **M**

LOSS OF APPETITE

Bay laurel, bergamot, caraway, cardomon, ginger, myrrh, black pepper.
Suggested application: **M**

NAUSEA/VOMITING

Allspice, lemon balm, French basil, cardomon, cascarilla bark, chamomile (German and Roman), clove bud, cilantro, sweet fennel, ginger, lavandin, lavender (spike and true), mint (peppermint and spearmint), nutmeg, black pepper, rose (cabbage and damask), rosewood, sandalwood.

FRESH PARSLEY

FRESH ALLSPICE

Suggested application:

M V

Genitourinary/Endocrine Systems

AMENORRHEA/LACK OF MENSTRUATION

French basil, bay laurel, carrot seed, celery seed, cinnamon leaf, dill, sweet fennel, hops, hyssop, juniper, lovage, sweet marjoram, myrrh, parsley, rose (cabbage and damask), sage (clary and Spanish), tarragon, yarrow.

Suggested application: **M B**

FRESH DILL

CYSTITIS

Canadian balsam, copaiba balsam, bergamot, cedarwood (Atlas, Texas, and Virginian), celery seed, chamomile (German and Roman), cubeb, blue gum eucalyptus, frankincense, juniper, lavandin, lavender (spike and true), lovage, mastic, niaouli, parsley, Scotch pine, sandalwood, tea tree, thyme, turpentine, yarrow.

Suggested application: **C B D**

DYSMENORRHEA/CRAMP, PAINFUL OR DIFFICULT MENSTRUATION

Lemon balm, French basil, carrot seed, chamomile (German and Roman), cypress, frankincense, hops, jasmine, juniper, lavandin, lavender (spike and true), lovage, sweet marjoram, rose (cabbage and damask), rosemary, sage (clary and Spanish), tarragon, yarrow.

Suggested application: **M C B**

FRIGIDITY

Cassie, cinnamon leaf, jasmine, nutmeg, orange blossom, parsley, patchouli, black pepper, cabbage rose, rosewood, clary sage, sandalwood, ylang ylang.

Suggested application: **M S B V**

LABOR PAIN AND CHILDBIRTH AID

Cinnamon leaf, jasmine, true lavender, nutmeg, parsley, rose (cabbage and damask), clary sage.

Suggested application: **M C B**

LACK OF NURSING MILK

Celery seed, dill, sweet fennel, hops.

Suggested application: **M**

LEUCORRHEA/WHITE DISCHARGE FROM THE VAGINA

Bergamot, cedarwood (Atlas, Texas, and Virginian), cinnamon leaf, cubeb, blue gum eucalyptus, frankincense, hyssop, lavandin, lavender (spike and true), sweet marjoram, mastic, myrrh, rosemary, clary sage, sandalwood, tea tree, turpentine.

Suggested application: **B D**

MENOPAUSAL PROBLEMS

Cypress, sweet fennel, geranium, jasmine, rose (cabbage and damask).

Suggested application: **M B V**

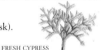

FRESH CYPRESS

MENORRHAGIA/EXCESSIVE MENSTRUATION

Chamomile (German and Roman), cypress, rose (cabbage and damask).

Suggested application: **M B**

PREMENSTRUAL SYNDROME/PMS

Carrot seed, chamomile (German and Roman), geranium, true lavender, sweet marjoram, orange blossom, tarragon.

Suggested application: **M B V**

PRURITIS/ITCHING

Bergamot, Atlas cedarwood, juniper, lavender, myrrh, tea tree.

Suggested application: **D**

FRESH JUNIPER

SEXUAL OVERACTIVITY

Hops, sweet marjoram.

Suggested application: **M B**

THRUSH/CANDIDA

Bergamot, geranium, myrrh, tea tree.

Suggested application: **B D**

URETHRITIS

Bergamot, cubeb, mastic, tea tree, turpentine.

Suggested application: **B D**

Immune System

CHICKENPOX

Bergamot, chamomile (German and Roman), eucalyptus (blue gum and lemon-scented), true lavender, tea tree. FRESH BERGAMOT
Suggested application: **C S B**

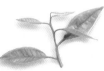

COLDS/FLU

Angelica, star anise, aniseed, copaiba balsam, Peru balsam, French basil, bay laurel, West Indian bay, bergamot, borneol, cabreuva, cajeput, camphor (white), caraway, cinnamon leaf, citronella, clove bud, cilantro, eucalyptus (blue gum, lemon-scented, and peppermint), silver fir, frankincense, ginger, grapefruit, helichrysum, juniper, lemon, lime, sweet marjoram, mastic, mint (peppermint and spearmint), myrtle, niaouli, orange (bitter and sweet), pine (longleaf and Scotch), rosemary, rosewood, Spanish sage, hemlock spruce, tea tree, thyme, turpentine, yarrow.
Suggested application: **M B V I**

HEMLOCK SPRUCE

FEVER

French basil, bergamot, borneol, camphor (white), eucalyptus (blue gum, lemon-scented, and peppermint), silver fir, ginger, helichrysum, juniper, lemon, lemongrass, lime, mint (peppermint and spearmint), myrtle, niaouli, rosemary, rosewood, Spanish sage, hemlock spruce, tea tree, thyme, yarrow.

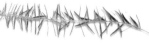

FRESH NIAOULI

Suggested application: **C B**

MEASLES

Bergamot, blue gum eucalyptus, lavender (spike and true), tea tree.
Suggested application: **S B I V**

Nervous System

ANXIETY

Ambrette, lemon balm, French basil, bergamot, cananga, frankincense, hyssop, jasmine, juniper, true lavender, mimosa, orange blossom, hemlock spruce, Levant styrax, lemon verbena, ylang ylang.
Suggested application:
M B V

LEVANT STYRAX

DEPRESSION

Allspice, ambrette, lemon balm, Canadian balsam, French basil, bergamot, cassie, grapefruit, helichrysum, jasmine, true lavender, orange blossom, rose (cabbage and damask), clary sage, sandalwood, hemlock spruce, vetiver, ylang ylang.
Suggested application: **M B V**

DRIED ROSE BUDS

HEADACHE

Chamomile (German and Roman), citronella, cumin, eucalyptus (blue gum and peppermint), grapefruit, hops, lavandin, lavender (spike and true), lemongrass, linden, sweet marjoram, mint (peppermint and spearmint), rose (cabbage and damask), rosemary, rosewood, sage (clary and Spanish), thyme, violet.
Suggested application: **M C V**

FRESH VIOLET

INSOMNIA

Lemon balm, French basil, calamintha, chamomile (German and Roman), hops, true lavender, linden, mandarin, sweet marjoram, orange blossom, petitgrain, rose (cabbage and damask), sandalwood, thyme, valerian, lemon verbena, vetiver, violet, yarrow, ylang ylang.
Suggested application: **M B V**

MIGRAINE

Angelica, lemon balm, French basil, chamomile (German and Roman), citronella, cilantro, true lavender, linden, sweet marjoram, mint (peppermint and spearmint), clary sage, valerian, yarrow. *Suggested application:* **C**

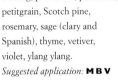

FRESH TRUE LAVENDER

NERVOUS EXHAUSTION OR FATIGUE/DEBILITY

Allspice, angelica, asafetida, French basil, borneol, cardomon, cassie, cinnamon leaf, citronella, cilantro, costus, cumin, elemi, eucalyptus (blue gum and peppermint), ginger, grapefruit, helichrysum, hyacinth, hyssop, jasmine, lavandin, spike lavender, lemongrass, mint (peppermint and spearmint), nutmeg, palmarosa, patchouli, petitgrain, Scotch pine, rosemary, sage (clary and Spanish), thyme, vetiver, violet, ylang ylang. *Suggested application:* **M B V**

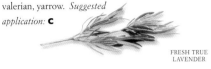

FRESH HELICHRYSUM

NERVOUS TENSION AND STRESS

Allspice, ambrette, angelica, asafetida, lemon balm, Canadian balsam, copaiba balsam, Peru balsam, French basil, benzoin, bergamot, borneol, calamintha, cananga, cardomon, cassie, cedarwood (Atlas, Texas, and Virginian), chamomile (German and Roman), cinnamon leaf, costus, cypress, elemi, frankincense, galbanum, geranium, helichrysum, hops, hyacinth, hyssop, jasmine, juniper, true lavender, lemongrass, linaloe, linden, mandarin, sweet marjoram, mimosa, mint

(peppermint and spearmint), orange (bitter and sweet), orange blossom, palmarosa, patchouli, petitgrain, Scotch pine, rose (cabbage and damask), rosemary, rosewood, clary sage, sandalwood, hemlock spruce, thyme, valerian, lemon verbena, vetiver, violet, yarrow, ylang ylang. *Suggested application:* **M B V**

FRESH LINDEN

NEURALGIA/SCIATICA

Allspice, West Indian bay, borneol, celery seed, chamomile (German and Roman), citronella, cilantro, eucalyptus (blue gum and peppermint), geranium, helichrysum, hops, spike lavender, sweet marjoram, mastic, mint (peppermint and spearmint), nutmeg, pine (longleaf and Scotch), rosemary, turpentine. *Suggested application:* **M B**

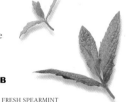

FRESH SPEARMINT

SHOCK

Lemon balm, lavandin, lavender (spike and true), orange blossom. *Suggested application:* **M B V**

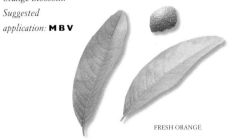

FRESH ORANGE

VERTIGO

Lemon balm, lavandin, lavender (spike and true), mint (peppermint and spearmint), violet. *Suggested application:* **V I**

The Oils

THE FOLLOWING PAGES *are a systematic survey of 167 essential oils, shown in alphabetical order according to the Latin name of the plants from which they are derived. The oils covered on these pages are all produced commercially, although some are little known or in scarce supply. A number of the oils have been designated as unsuitable for therapeutic use but have been included in this section for two reasons: first, to present a comprehensive picture of all the essential oils that are readily available; and second, to inform the reader about the possible dangers of such oils.*

BLENDED
OIL

Aromatic plants are found all over the world, and essential oil production is an international industry, of which the "aromatherapy market" plays a small but rapidly expanding part. Individual entries contain a general description of the plant (illustrated in each case), the most up-to-date information about the actions of each essential oil, the methods of extraction, compatibilities with other oils (where relevant), a detailed guide to home and commercial uses, and safety data.

SPEARMINT

BERGAMOT
SPRIG

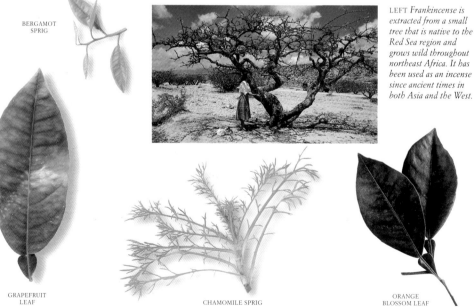

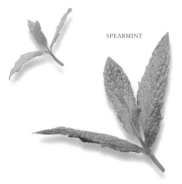

LEFT *Frankincense is extracted from a small tree that is native to the Red Sea region and grows wild throughout northeast Africa. It has been used as an incense since ancient times in both Asia and the West.*

GRAPEFRUIT
LEAF

CHAMOMILE SPRIG

ORANGE
BLOSSOM LEAF

ABELMOSCHUS MOSCHATUS

Ambrette seed

FAMILY: MALVACEAE

Herbal/Folk Tradition
Generally used as a stimulant and to ease indigestion, cramp, and nervous dyspepsia. Widely used as a domestic spice in the East. In China it is used to treat headaches; in Egypt the seeds are used to sweeten the breath.

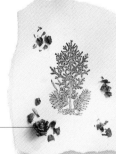

SEEDS

An evergreen shrub about 5ft (1.5m) high, bearing large single yellow flowers with purple centers. The capsules, in the form of five-cornered pyramids, contain grayish-brown, kidney-shaped seeds that have a musky odor.

DATAFILE

AROMATHERAPY/ HOME USE
Circulation, Muscles, and Joints: *Cramp, fatigue, muscular aches and pains, poor circulation.*
Nervous System: *Anxiety, depression, nervous tension, and stress-related conditions.*

EXTRACTION
Essential oil by steam distillation of the seeds. Liquid ambrette seed should be allowed to age for several months before it is used. A concrete and absolute are also produced by solvent extraction.

ACTIONS
Antispasmodic, aphrodisiac, carminative, nervine, stimulant, stomachic.

COMPATIBILITIES
It blends well with rose, orange blossom, sandalwood, clary sage, cypress, patchouli, oriental, and "sophisticated" bases.

SAFETY DATA
Nontoxic, nonirritant, and nonsensitizing

ABIES ALBA

Silver fir needle

FAMILY: PINACEAE

Herbal/Folk Tradition
It is highly esteemed in Europe for its medicinal virtues and its fragrant scent. It is used mainly for respiratory complaints, fever, muscular and rheumatic pain.

SILVER FIR CONE

A relatively small coniferous tree, with a regular pyramidal shape and a silvery white bark, grown chiefly for lumber and as Christmas trees.

DATAFILE

AROMATHERAPY/ HOME USE
Circulation, Muscles, and Joints: *Arthritis, muscular aches and pains, rheumatism.*
Respiratory System: *Bronchitis, coughs, sinusitis, etc.*
Immune System: *Colds, fever, flu.*

EXTRACTION
Essential oil by steam distillation from needles and young twigs, and from broken-up fir cones,

ACTIONS
Analgesic, antiseptic (pulmonary), antitussive, deodorant, expectorant, rubefacient, stimulant, tonic.

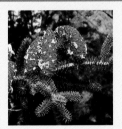

Abies alba

COMPATIBILITIES
It blends well with galbanum, labdanum, lavender, rosemary, lemon, pine, and marjoram.

SAFETY DATA
Nontoxic, nonirritant (except in high concentration), nonsensitizing

ABIES BALSAMEA

Canadian balsam

FAMILY: PINACEAE

Herbal/Folk Tradition

The oleoresin is used extensively by Native Americans for ritual purposes and as an external treatment for burns, sores, cuts, and to relieve heart and chest pains. It is also used internally for coughs.

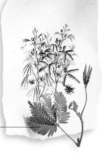

DRIED CANADIAN BALSAM

An evergreen tree up to 65ft (20m) high, with a tapering trunk and numerous branches, creating the overall shape of a perfect cone. It forms blisters of oleoresin (the so-called balsam) on the trunk and branches.

DATAFILE

AROMATHERAPY/ HOME USE
Skin Care: *Burns, cuts, hemorrhoids, wounds.*
Respiratory System: *Asthma, bronchitis, catarrh, chronic coughs, sore throat.*
Genitourinary System: *Cystitis, genitourinary infections.*
Nervous System: *Depression, nervous tension, stress-related conditions.*

EXTRACTION
The oleoresin is collected by puncturing vesicles in the bark. An essential oil is produced by steam distillation from the oleoresin (Canada balsam or Canada turpentine). Fir needle oil is produced by steam distillation from the leaf or needles.

ACTIONS
Antiseptic (genitourinary, pulmonary), antitussive, astringent, cicatrizant, diuretic, expectorant, purgative, regulatory, sedative (nerve), tonic, vulnerary.

COMPATIBILITIES
It blends well with pine, cypress, sandalwood, juniper, benzoin, and other balsams.

SAFETY DATA
Generally nontoxic, nonirritant, nonsensitizing

ACACIA DEALBATA

Mimosa

FAMILY: MIMOSACEAE

Herbal/Folk Tradition

The bark of mimosa ("wattle bark") has a leatherlike odor and astringent taste. It contains up to 42 per cent tannins (also gallic acid) and is used as a specific for diarrhea, and as an astringent gargle and ointment.

FRESH MIMOSA

An attractive small tree up to 39ft (12m) high, having a grayish-brown bark with irregular, longitudinal ridges, delicate foliage, and clusters of fragrant yellow flowers.

DATAFILE

AROMATHERAPY/ HOME USE
Skin Care: *Oily, sensitive, general skin care.*
Nervous System: *Anxiety, nervous tension, oversensitivity, stress.*

EXTRACTION
A concrete and absolute by solvent extraction from the flowers and twig ends,

ACTIONS
Antiseptic, astringent.

COMPATIBILITIES
It blends well with lavandin, lavender, ylang, ylang, violet, styrax, cironella, Peru balsam,

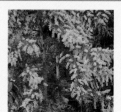

Acacia dealbata

cassie, floral and spice oils. It is employed largely in soaps and also in high-quality perfumes, especially colognes, floral and oriental types.

SAFETY DATA
Nontoxic, nonirritant, nonsensitizing

ACACIA FARNESIANA

Cassie

FAMILY: MIMOSACEAE

Herbal/Folk Tradition

In India "attar of cassie" is made as a perfume. The fresh flowers are used in baths for dry skin. In Venezuela the root is used to treat stomach cancer. In China it is used to treat rheumatoid arthritis and pulmonary tuberculosis.

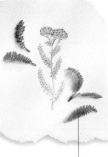

DRIED FLOWERS

A bushy, thorny shrub, much branched, up to 33ft (10m) high. It has a very delicate appearance, similar to mimosa, with fragrant fluffy yellow flowers.

DATAFILE

AROMATHERAPY/HOME USE
Use with care for:
Skin Care: *Dry, sensitive skin, perfume.*
Nervous System: *Depression, frigidity, nervous exhaustion, and stress-related conditions.*

EXTRACTION
An absolute by solvent extraction from the flowers.

ACTIONS
Antirheumatic, antiseptic, antispasmodic, aphrodisiac, balsamic, insecticide.

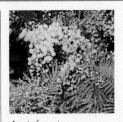

Acacia farnesiana

COMPATIBILITIES
It blends well with bergamot, costus, mimosa, frankincense, ylang ylang, orris, and violet and is used in high-quality perfumes, especially oriental types.

SAFETY DATA
No available data on toxicity

ACHILLEA MILLEFOLIUM

Yarrow

FAMILY: ASTERACEAE (COMPOSITAE)

Herbal/Folk Tradition

An age-old herbal medicine used for a wide variety of complaints including fever, respiratory infections, digestive problems, nervous tension, and externally for sores, rashes, and wounds.

FRESH YARROW

A perennial herb with a simple stem up to 3ft (1m) high, with finely dissected leaves giving a lacy appearance, bearing numerous pinky-white, dense flowerheads.

DATAFILE

AROMATHERAPY/HOME USE
Skin Care: *Acne, burns, cuts, eczema, hair rinse (promotes hair growth), inflammations, rashes, scars, varicose veins, wounds.*
Circulation, Muscles, and Joints: *Arteriosclerosis, high blood pressure, rheumatoid arthritis, thrombosis.*
Digestive System: *Constipation, cramp, flatulence, hemorrhoids, indigestion.*
Genitourinary System: *Amenorrhea, dysmenorrhea, cystitis, and other infections.*
Immune System: *Colds, fever, flu.*
Nervous System: *Hypertension, insomnia, stress.*

EXTRACTION
Essential oil by steam distillation from the dried herb.

ACTIONS
Anti-inflammatory, antipyretic, antirheumatic, antiseptic, antispasmodic, astringent, carminative, cicatrisant, diaphoretic, digestive, expectorant, hemostatic, hypotensive, stomachic, tonic.

COMPATIBILITIES
It blends well with cedarwood, pine, chamomile, valerian, vetiver, and oakmoss.

SAFETY DATA
Non-toxic, non-irritant, possible sensitization in some individuals

45

ACORUS CALAMUS VAR. ANGUSTATUS

Calamus

FAMILY: ARACEAE

Herbal/Folk Tradition

FRESH CALAMUS

The aromatic oil, contained largely in the root, used to be highly esteemed as an aromatic stimulant and tonic for fever (typhoid), nervous complaints, vertigo, headaches, and dysentery.

CALAMUS ROOT

A reedlike aquatic plant about 3ft (1m) high, with sword-shaped leaves and small greenish-yellow flowers. It grows on the margins of lakes and streams with the long-branched rhizome immersed in the mud.

DATAFILE

AROMATHERAPY/ HOME USE
None. "Should not be used in therapy, whether internally or externally."[2] It is extensively used in cosmetic and perfumery work, in woody/oriental/leather perfumes and to scent hair and tooth powders.

EXTRACTION
Essential oil by steam distillation from the rhizomes (and sometimes the leaves).

ACTIONS
Anticonvulsant, antiseptic, bactericidal, carminative, diaphoretic, expectorant,

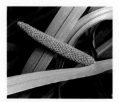

Acorus calamus var. angustatus

hypotensive, insecticide, spasmolytic, stimulant, stomachic, tonic, vermifuge.

COMPATIBILITIES
It blends well with cananga, cinnamon, labdanum, olibanum, patchouli, cedarwood, amyris, spice and oriental bases.

SAFETY DATA
Oral toxin. The oil of calamus is reported to have carcinogenic properties

AGOTHOSMA BETULINA

Buchu

FAMILY: RUTACEAE

Herbal/Folk Tradition

The leaves are used locally as an antiseptic and to ward off insects. In the West, the leaves are used for infections of the genitourinary system.

FRESH AND
DRIED BUCHU

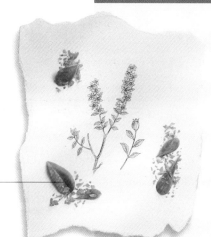

A small, aromatic shrub with simple wrinkled leaves about ½in (1–2cm) long; other much smaller leaves are also present, which are bright green with finely serrated margins. Its delicate stems bear five-petaled white flowers.

DATAFILE

AROMATHERAPY/ HOME USE
None. A tincture, extract, and oleoresin are produced for pharmaceutical use. Limited use in blackcurrant flavor and fragrance work, for example, colognes and chypré bases.

EXTRACTION
Essential oil by steam distillation from the dried leaves.

ACTIONS
Antiseptic (especially urinary), carminative, diaphoretic, diuretic, insecticide, stimulant, tonic.

SAFETY DATA
Should not be used during pregnancy

ALLIUM CEPA

Onion

FAMILY: LILIACEAE

Herbal/Folk Tradition

Onion has an ancient reputation as a curative agent. It is high in vitamins A, B, and C. Raw onion helps to keep infections and colds at bay, promotes strong bones, and a good blood supply. It is an effective blood cleanser and keeps the skin clear.

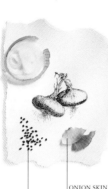

ONION SKIN

ONION SEED

A perennial or biennial herb up to 4ft (1.2m) high with hollow leaves and flowering stem, and a globelike, fleshy bulb.

DATAFILE

AROMATHERAPY/ HOME USE

None, due to its offensive, sulfuraceous smell. It is, however, used in some pharmaceutical preparations for colds, coughs, etc. The oil is used extensively in most major food categories, especially meats, savories, and salad dressings.

EXTRACTION

Essential oil by steam distillation from the bulb. (An oleoresin is also produced in small quantities for flavoring use).

ACTIONS

Anthelmintic, antimicrobial, antirheumatic, antiseptic, antisclerotic, antispasmodic, antiviral, bactericidal, carminative, depurative, digestive, diuretic, expectorant, fungicidal, hypocholesterolemic, hypoglycemic, hypotensive, stomachic, tonic, vermifuge.

SAFETY DATA

Specific safety data unavailable at present – probably similar to garlic, i.e. generally nontoxic, nonirritant, possible sensitization

---

ALLIUM SATIVUM

Garlic

FAMILY: AMARYLLIDACEAE OR LILIACEAE

Herbal/Folk Tradition

Used for thousands of years for respiratory and urinary tract infections, digestive problems, heart disease, high blood pressure, epidemics and fever.

GARLIC BULB

CLOVE OF GARLIC

A strongly scented perennial herb up to 4ft (1.2m) high with long, flat, firm leaves and whitish flowering stems. The bulb is made up of several cloves pressed together within a thin white skin.

DATAFILE

AROMATHERAPY/ HOME USE

Due to its unpleasant and pervasive smell, the oil is not often used externally. However, the capsules may be taken internally according to the instructions on the label for respiratory and gastrointestinal infections, urinary tract infections such as cystitis, heart and circulatory problems, and to fight infectious diseases in general.

EXTRACTION

Essential oil by steam distillation from the fresh crushed bulbs.

ACTIONS

Amoebicidal, anthelmintic, antibiotic, antimicrobial, antiseptic, antitoxic, antitumor, antiviral, bactericidal, carminative, cholagogue, hypocholesterolemic, depurative, diaphoretic, diuretic, expectorant, febrifuge, fungicidal, hypoglycemic, hypotensive, insecticidal, larvicidal, promotes leucocytosis, stomachic, tonic.

SAFETY DATA

Generally nontoxic and nonirritant, although it has been known to irritate the stomach; may also cause sensitization in some individuals

ALOYSIA TRIPHYLLA

Lemon verbena

FAMILY: VERBENACEAE

Herbal/Folk Tradition

Lemon verbena is indicated especially in nervous conditions that manifest as digestive complaints. The dried leaves are used as a tea, both as a refreshing "pick-me-up" and to help restore the liver after a hangover.

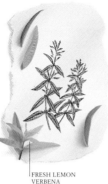

FRESH LEMON VERBENA

A handsome deciduous perennial shrub up to 16ft (5m) high with a woody stem, very fragrant, delicate, pale green, lanceolate leaves arranged in threes, and small, pale purple flowers. Often grown as an ornamental bush.

DATAFILE

AROMATHERAPY/ HOME USE
Digestive System: *Cramps, indigestion, liver congestion.*
Nervous System: *Anxiety, insomnia, nervous tension, and stress-related conditions.*
True verbena oil is virtually non-existent. Most so-called verbena oil is either from the Spanish verbena (an inferior oil) or a mix of lemongrass, lemon, citronella, etc.

EXTRACTION
Essential oil by steam distillation from the freshly harvested herb.

ACTIONS
Antiseptic, antispasmodic, carminative, detoxifying, digestive, febrifuge, hepatobiliary stimulant, sedative (nervous), stomachic.

COMPATIBILITIES
It blends well with neroli, palmarosa, olibanum, Tolu balsam, elemi, lemon, and other citrus oils.

SAFETY DATA
Possible sensitization; phototoxicity due to high citral levels. Other saftey data is unavailable at present

---

ALPINIA OFFICINARUM

Galangal

FAMILY: ZINGIBERACEA

Herbal/Folk Tradition

It is used as a local spice, especially in curries; in India it is employed in perfumery. The root is current in the British Herbal Pharmacopoeia, indicated for dyspepsia, flatulence, colic, nausea, and vomiting.

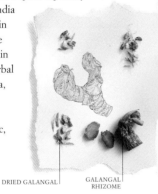

DRIED GALANGAL | GALANGAL RHIZOME

A reedlike plant reaching a height of about 3ft (1m), with irregularly branched rhizomes red or brown on the outside, light orange within.

DATAFILE

AROMATHERAPY/ HOME USE
(Possibly digestive upsets.) It is also used as a flavor ingredient, especially in spice and meat products, and is occasionally used in perfumery.

EXTRACTION
Essential oil by steam distillation from the rhizomes. (An oleoresin is also produced by solvent extraction.)

ACTIONS
Antiseptic, bactericidal, carminative, diaphoretic, stimulant, stomachic.

COMPATIBILITIES
It blends well with chamomile maroc, sage, cinnamon, allspice, lavandin, pine needle, rosemary, patchouli, myrtle, opopanax, and citrus oils.

SAFETY DATA
Safety data unavailable at present

AMYRIS BALSAMIFERA

Amyris

FAMILY: RUTACEAE

AMYRIS CHIPPINGS

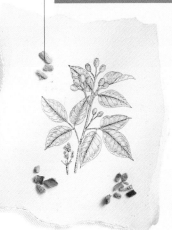

Herbal/Folk Tradition
Locals call this bushy tree, which originated in Haiti and is cultivated in tropical zones all over the world, "candle wood" because of its high oil content; it burns like a candle. It is used as a torch by fishermen and traders. It also makes excellent furniture wood.

A small bushy tree with compound leaves and white flowers, which grows wild in thickets all over the island of Haiti.

DATAFILE

AROMATHERAPY/ HOME USE
Perfume.

EXTRACTION
Essential oil by steam distillation from the broken-up wood and branches. Best if the wood is seasoned first. It provides a very plentiful yield.

ACTIONS
Antiseptic, balsamic, sedative.

COMPATIBILITIES
It blends well with lavandin, citronella, oakmoss, sassafras, cedarwood, and wood oils.

SAFETY DATA
Nontoxic, nonirritant, nonsensitizing

ANETHUM GRAVEOLENS

Dill

FAMILY: APIACEAE (UMBELLIFERAE)

Herbal/Folk Tradition
Used since the earliest times as a medicinal and culinary herb, especially in Germany and Scandinavia. In the West and East it is used as a digestive aid for indigestion, wind, colic, etc., especially in children.

FRESH DILL

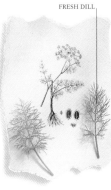

Annual or biennial herb up to 3ft (1m) high with a smooth stem, feathery leaves and umbels of yellowish flowers followed by flat, small seeds.

DATAFILE

AROMATHERAPY/ HOME USE
Digestive System: *Colic, dyspepsia, flatulence, indigestion.* Genitourinary and Endocrine Systems: *Lack of periods; promotes milk flow in nursing mothers.*

EXTRACTION
Essential oil by steam distillation from fruit or seed, and herb or weed (fresh or partially dried).

ACTIONS
Antispasmodic, bactericidal, carminative, digestive, emmenagogue, galactagogue, hypotensive, stimulant, stomachic.

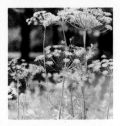

Anethum graveolens

COMPATIBILITIES
It blends well with elemi, mint, caraway, nutmeg, and spice and citrus oils.

SAFETY DATA
Nontoxic, nonirritant, nonsensitizing

49

ANGELICA ARCHANGELICA

Angelica

FAMILY: APIACEAE (UMBELLIFERAE)

Herbal/Folk Tradition

This herb has been praised for its virtues since antiquity. It strengthens the heart, stimulates the circulation and the immune system. It is used for rheumatic inflammation, bronchial ailments, colds, indigestion, wind, and as an appetite stimulant and urinary antiseptic.

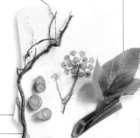

FRESH ANGELICA

SECTION OF
FRESH STALK

ANGELICA ROOT

A large, hairy plant with ferny leaves and umbels of white flowers. It has a strong aromatic scent and a large rhizome.

DATAFILE

**AROMATHERAPY/
HOME USE**
Skin Care: *Dull congested skin, irritated conditions, psoriasis.*
Circulation, Muscles, and Joints: *Accumulation of toxins, arthritis, gout, rheumatism, water retention.*
Respiratory System: *Bronchitis, coughs.*
Digestive System: *Anemia, anorexia, flatulence, indigestion.*
Nervous System: *Fatigue, migraine, nervous tension, and stress-related disorders.*
Immune System: *Colds.*

EXTRACTION
Essential oil produced by steam distillation from the roots and rhizomes, and fruit or seed.

ACTIONS
Antispasmodic, carminative, depurative, diaphoretic, digestive, diuretic, emmenagogue, expectorant, febrifuge, nervine, stimulant, stomachic, tonic.

COMPATIBILITIES
It blends well with patchouli, opopanax, costus, clary sage, oakmoss, veitiver, and citrus oils.

SAFETY DATA
Both root and seed oil are nontoxic and nonirritant. The root oil (not the seed oil) is phototoxic, probably due to higher levels of bergapten. Not to be used during pregnancy or by diabetics

---

ANIBA ROSAEODORA

Rosewood

FAMILY: LAURACEAE

Herbal/Folk Tradition

Used for building, carving, and French cabinet-making. Nowadays, most rosewood goes to Japan for the production of chopsticks.

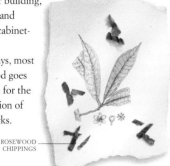

ROSEWOOD
CHIPPINGS

Medium-size, tropical, evergreen tree with a reddish bark and heartwood, bearing yellow flowers. Used extensively for lumber. NB: Rosewood is being extensively felled in the clearing of the South American rainforests; the production of rosewood oil is consequently environmentally damaging.

DATAFILE

**AROMATHERAPY/
HOME USE**
Skin Care: *Acne, dermatitis, scars, wounds, wrinkles, and general skin care: sensitive, dry, dull, combination oily/dry, etc. "Although it does not have any dramatic curative power . I find it very useful especially for skin care. It is very mild and safe to use."*[3]
Immune System: *Colds, coughs, fever, infections, stimulates the immune system.*
Nervous System: *Frigidity, headaches, nausea, nervous tension, and stress-related conditions.*

EXTRACTION
Essential oil by steam distillation of the wood chippings.

ACTIONS
Mildly analgesic, anticonvulsant, antidepressant, antimicrobial, antiseptic, aphrodisiac, bactericidal, cellular stimulant, cephalic, deodorant, stimulant (immune system), tissue regenerator, tonic.

COMPATIBILITIES
It blends well with most oils, especially citrus, woods, and florals. It helps give body and rounds off sharp edges.

SAFETY DATA
Nontoxic, nonirritant, nonsensitizing

ANTHRISCUS CEREFOLIUM

Chervil

FAMILY: APIACEAE (UMBELLIFERAE)

Herbal/Folk Tradition

The leaves are used as a domestic spice. In folk medicine it is used as a tea to tone up the blood and nerves, and for poor memory and depression. Juice is used for skin ailments such as eczema, abscesses, and slow-healing wounds.

SPRIG OF FRESH CHERVIL

An annual herb up to 12in (30cm) high, with a slender, much-branched stem, bright green, finely divided, fernlike leaves, umbels of flat white flowerheads and long smooth seeds or fruits. It has an aromatic scent when bruised.

DATAFILE

AROMATHERAPY/ HOME USE
None. Methyl chavicol and anethole are known to have toxic and irritant effects; methyl chavicol is reported to have possible carcinogenic effects. Since these constitute the major proportion of the essential oil, it is best avoided for therapeutic use.

EXTRACTION
Essential oil by steam distillation from seeds or fruit

ACTIONS
Aperitif, antiseptic, carminative, cicatrisant, depurative, diaphoretic, digestive, diuretic, nervine, restorative, stimulant (metabolism), stomachic, tonic.

Anthriscus cerefolium

SAFETY DATA
Toxic and irritant effects; possibly carcinogenic effects

APIUM GRAVEOLENS

Celery seed

FAMILY: APIACEAE (UMBELLIFERAE)

Herbal/Folk Tradition

The seed is used in bladder and kidney complaints, digestive upsets, and menstrual problems; the leaves are used in skin ailments. It is known to increase the elimination of uric acid and is useful for gout, neuralgia, and rheumatoid arthritis.

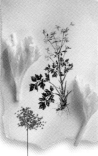

CELERY SEED

A familiar biennial plant, 12–24in (30–60cm) high, with a grooved, fleshy, erect stalk, shiny pinnate leaves, and umbels of white flowers.

DATAFILE

AROMATHERAPY/ HOME USE
Circulation, Muscles, and Joints: *Arthritis, buildup of toxins in the blood, gout, rheumatism.*
Digestive System: *Dyspepsia, flatulence, indigestion, liver congestion, jaundice.*
Genitourinary and Endocrine Systems: *Amenorrhea, glandular problems, increases milk flow, cystitis.*
Nervous System: *Neuralgia, sciatica.*

EXTRACTION
Essential oil by steam distillation from whole or crushed seeds. An oil from the whole herb; an oleoresin, and extract are also produced in small quantities.

ACTIONS
Antioxidative, antirheumatic, antiseptic (urinary), antispasmodic, aperitif, depurative, digestive, diuretic, carminative, cholagogue, emmenagogue, galactagogue, hepatic, nervine, sedative (nervous), stimulant (uterine), stomachic, tonic (digestive).

COMPATIBILITIES
It blends well with lavender, pine, opopanax, lovage, tea tree, oakmoss, cilantro, and other spices.

SAFETY DATA
Nontoxic, nonirritant, possible sensitization. Avoid during pregnancy

ARMORACIA RUSTICANA

Horseradish

FAMILY: BRASSICACEAE (CRUCIFERAE)

Herbal/Folk Tradition

An extremely
stimulating herb,
once valued as a
household
remedy. It was
used for fever,
digestive
complaints,
urinary
infections, and
as a circulatory
aid. Good for arthritis
and rheumatism.

HORSERADISH
ROOT

SECTION OF ROOT

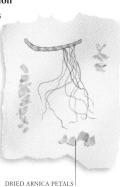

*A perennial plant with large leaves up to 20in (50cm) long,
white flowers, and a thick, whitish, tapering root, which is
propagated easily.*

**AROMATHERAPY/
HOME USE**
None. This essential oil should
not be used in therapy either
externally or internally. It is
used mainly in minute amounts
in seasonings, ready-made
salads, condiments, and canned
products.

EXTRACTION
Essential oil by water and steam
distillation from the broken
roots that have been soaked in
water. (A resinoid or concrete
is also produced by solvent
extraction.)

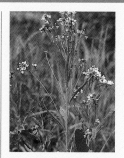

Armoracia rusticana

ACTIONS
Antibiotic, antiseptic, diuretic,
carminative, expectorant,
laxative (mild), rubefacient,
stimulant.

SAFETY DATA
Oral toxin, dermal irritant, mucous membrane irritant

ARNICA MONTANA

Arnica

FAMILY: ASTERACEAE (COMPOSITAE)

Herbal/Folk Tradition

This herb stimulates
the peripheral
blood supply
when applied
externally, and
is one of the
best remedies
for bruises and
sprains. It is
never used
internally.

DRIED ARNICA PETALS

*A perennial alpine herb with a creeping underground stem,
giving rise to a rosette of pale oval leaves. The flowering,
erect stem is up to 24in (60cm) high, bearing a single, bright
yellow, daisylike flower. The plant is difficult to cultivate.*

**AROMATHERAPY/
HOME USE**
None.

EXTRACTION
Essential oil by steam distillation
of flowers and root. The yield of
essential oil is very small. An
absolute, tincture, and resinoid
are also produced.

ACTIONS
Anti-inflammatory, stimulant,
vulnerary.

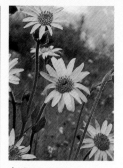

*Arnica montana
Native to northern and central
Europe, also found growing
wild in Russia, Scandinavia,
and northern India.*

SAFETY DATA
*The essential oil is highly toxic and should never be used internally
or on broken skin. However, the tincture or arnica ointment are
valuable additions to the home medicine cabinet*

ARTEMISIA ABSINTHIUM

Wormwood

FAMILY: ASTERACEAE (COMPOSITAE)

Herbal/Folk Tradition

Used as an aromatic-bitter for anorexia, as a digestive tonic, and as a choleretic for liver and gall bladder disorders, usually in the form of a dilute extract. It is also used to promote menstruation, reduce fever, and expel worms.

FRESH WORMWOOD

A perennial herb up to 5ft (1.5m) high with a whitish stem, silvery-green, divided leaves covered with silky, fine hairs, and pale yellow flowers.

DATAFILE

AROMATHERAPY/ HOME USE
None. This oil should not be used in therapy. Habitual use can cause restlessness, nightmares, convulsions, vomiting, and, in extreme cases, brain damage. In 1915 the French banned the production of the drink absinthe with this plant, because of its narcotic and habit-forming properties.

EXTRACTION
Essential oil by steam distillation from the leaves and flowering tops. (An absolute is occasionally produced by solvent extraction.)

ACTIONS
Anthelmintic, choleretic, deodorant, emmenagogue, febrifuge, insect repellant, narcotic, stimulant (digestive), tonic, vermifuge.

COMPATIBILITIES
It blends well with oakmoss, jasmine, orange blossom, lavender, and hyacinth.

SAFETY DATA
Toxic. Abortifacient

ARTEMISIA DRACUNCULUS

Tarragon

FAMILY: ASTERCEAE (COMPOSITAE)

Herbal/Folk Tradition

The leaf is commonly used as a domestic herb and to make tarragon vinegar. The maharajahs of India took it as a tisane, and in Persia it was used to induce appetite. The leaf was also used for digestive and menstrual irregularities.

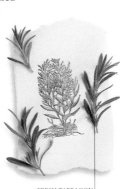

FRESH TARRAGON

A perennial herb with smooth narrow leaves; an erect stem up to 1.2m (4ft) tall, and small yellowy-green, inconspicuous flowers.

DATAFILE

AROMATHERAPY/ HOME USE
Digestive System: *Anorexia, dyspepsia, flatulence, hiccoughs, intestinal spasm, nervous indigestion, sluggish digestion.*
Genitourinary System: *Amenorrhea, dysmenorrhea, PMS.*

EXTRACTION
Essential oil by steam distillation from the leaves.

ACTIONS
Anthelmintic, antiseptic, antispasmodic, aperitif, carminative, digestive, diuretic, emmenagogue, hypnotic, stimulant, stomachic, vermifuge.

COMPATIBILITIES
It blends well with labdanum, galbanum, lavender, oakmoss, vanilla, pine, and basil.

SAFETY DATA
Moderately toxic due to "estragole" (methyl chavicol): use in moderation only. Possibly carcinogenic. Otherwise nonirritant, nonsensitizing. Avoid during pregnancy

ARTEMISIA VULGARIS

Mugwort

FAMILY: ASTERACEAE (COMPOSITAE)

Herbal/Folk Tradition

Associated, in Europe, with witchcraft and superstition. It was seen as a woman's plant, used as a womb tonic, for painful, delayed menstruation, and for hysteria and epilepsy. It was also used to expel worms, control fever, and as a digestive remedy.

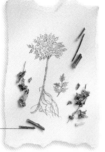

DRIED MUGWORT LEAVES

An erect, much-branched, perennial herb up to 5ft (1.5m) high, with purplish stems, dark green divided leaves that are downy white beneath, and numerous small reddish-brown or yellow flowers.

DATAFILE

AROMATHERAPY/ HOME USE
None. It should not be used in therapy either internally or externally. It is, however, used as a fragrance component in soaps, colognes, and perfumes.

EXTRACTION
Essential oil by steam distillation from the leaves and flowering tops.

ACTIONS
Anthelmintic, antispasmodic, carminative, choleretic, diaphoretic, diuretic, emmenagogue, nervine, orexigenic, stimulant, stomachic, tonic (uterine, womb), vermifuge.

COMPATIBILITIES
It blends well with oakmoss, patchouli, rosemary, lavandin, pine, sage, clary sage, and cedarwood.

SAFETY DATA
Oral toxin, due to high thujone content. Abortifacient

ASARUM CANADENSE

Snakeroot

FAMILY: ARISTOLOCHIACEAE

Herbal/Folk Tradition

This plant has been used for centuries in folk medicine but is now little prescribed. It was used for chronic chest complaints, rheumatism, dropsy, and painful bowel and stomach spasms.

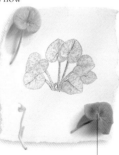

FRESH SNAKEROOT

A fragrant little plant not more than 14in (35cm) high with hairy stem, two glossy, kidney-shaped leaves, and a creeping rootstock. The solitary bell-shaped flower is brownish purple, and creamy white inside.

DATAFILE

AROMATHERAPY/ HOME USE
May possibly be used for its antispasmodic qualities, for example, for period pains or indigestion.

EXTRACTION
Essential oil by steam distillation from dried rhizomes and crushed roots.

ACTIONS
Anti-inflammatory, antispasmodic, carminative, diuretic, diaphoretic, emmenagogue, expectorant, febrifuge, stimulant, stomachic.

COMPATIBILITIES
It blends well with bergamot, costus, oakmoss, patchouli, pine needle, clary sage, mimosa, cassie, and other florals.

SAFETY DATA
Nontoxic, nonirritant, nonsensitizing. Avoid during pregnancy

BETULA ALBA

White birch

FAMILY: BETULACEAE

Herbal/Folk Tradition

Birch buds were formerly used as a tonic in hair preparations. Birch tar is used in Europe for chronic skin complaints, such as psoriasis, eczema. In Scandinavia the sap is tapped and drunk as a tonic, and birch leaflets and twigs are used in the sauna.

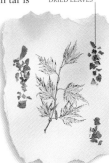

DRIED LEAVES

Decorative tree, up to 49–65ft (15–20m) high, with slender branches, silvery-white bark broken into scales, and light green oval leaves. The male catkins are 1–2in (2–5cm) long, the female up to 6in (15cm) long.

DATAFILE

AROMATHERAPY/ HOME USE

Skin Care: *Dermatitis, dull or congested skin, eczema, hair care, psoriasis, etc.*

Circulation, Muscles, and Joints: *Accumulation of toxins, arthritis, cellulitis, muscular pain, obesity, edema, poor circulation, rheumatism.*

EXTRACTION
Essential oil by steam distillation from the leaf-buds. Crude birch tar is also extracted by slow destructive distillation from the bark; this is subsequently steam-distilled to yield a rectified birch tar oil.

ACTIONS
Anti-inflammatory, antiseptic, cholagogue, diaphoretic, diuretic, febrifuge, tonic.

COMPATIBILITIES
It blends well with other woody and balsamic oils.

SAFETY DATA
Nontoxic, nonirritant, nonsensitizing

BETULA LENTA

Sweet birch

FAMILY: BETULACEAE

Herbal/Folk Tradition

The cambium (the layer directly under the bark) is eaten in the spring. Bark infusion is used as a stimulant and to promote sweating. As a decoction or syrup, it is used as a tonic for dysentery.

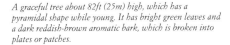

AROMATIC BARK

A SPRIG OF
SWEET BIRCH

A graceful tree about 82ft (25m) high, which has a pyramidal shape while young. It has bright green leaves and a dark reddish-brown aromatic bark, which is broken into plates or patches.

DATAFILE

AROMATHERAPY/ HOME USE

None. Methyl salicylate can be absorbed through the skin, and can cause fatal poisoning. It is also classed as an environmental hazard or marine pollutant.

EXTRACTION
Essential oil by steam distillation of the bark macerated in water.

ACTIONS
Analgesic, anti-inflammatory, antipyretic, antirheumatic, antiseptic, astringent, depurative, diuretic, rubefacient, tonic.

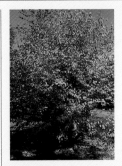

*Betula lenta
Native to southern Canada and eastern United States. Produced mainly in Pennsylvania.*

SAFETY DATA
Methyl salicylate, the major constituent, is not exactly toxic but very harmful in concentration

BORONIA MEGASTIGMA

Boronia

FAMILY: RUTACEAE

Herbal/Folk Tradition

A botanist in the Victorian era suggested this species would be suitable for graveyard planting because of its dark flowers!

DRIED FLOWERS

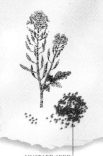

A bushy evergreen shrub, up to 6ft (2m) high, which bears an abundance of fragrant, nodding flowers with an unusual coloring – the petals are brown on the outside, yellow on the inside. Often grown as an ornamental shrub in gardens.

AROMATHERAPY/ HOME USE
Perfume.

EXTRACTION
A concrete and absolute by the enfleurage method or petroleum-ether extraction, from the flowers. Essential oil is by steam distillation.

ACTIONS
Aromatic.

COMPATIBILITIES
It blends well with clary sage, sandalwood, bergamot, violet, helichrysum, costus, mimosa, and other florals.

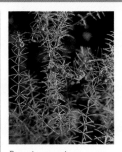

Boronia megastigma
Native to Western Australia; grows wild all over west and southwest Australia.

SAFETY DATA
Prohibitively expensive and therefore often adulterated

BRASSICA NIGRA

Mustard

FAMILY: BRASSICACEAE (CRUCIFERAE)

Herbal/Folk Tradition

The seeds are highly esteemed as a condiment and for their medicinal qualities. Used to aid digestion, and promote the appetite, and for colds, chills, coughs, chilblains, rheumatism, arthritis, lumbago, and aches and pains.

MUSTARD SEED

An erect annual up to 10ft (3m) high, with spear-shaped upper leaves, smooth flat pods containing about ten dark brown seeds, and yellow flowers.

AROMATHERAPY/ HOME USE
None. It is not recommended for therapy, either externally or internally.

EXTRACTION
Essential oil by steam (or water) distillation from the black mustard seeds, which have been macerated in warm water.

ACTIONS
Aperitif, antimicrobial, antiseptic, diuretic, emetic, febrifuge, rubefacient (produces blistering of the skin), stimulant.

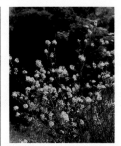

Brassica nigra
Common throughout eastern Europe, southern Siberia, Asia Minor, and North Africa; naturalized in North and South America.

SAFETY DATA
Oral toxin, dermal toxin, mucous membrane irritant. It is considered one of the most toxic of all essential oils

BOSWELLIA CARTERI

Frankincense

FAMILY: BURSERACEA

Herbal/Folk Tradition

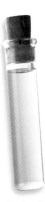

Used since antiquity as an incense in India, China, and in the West by the Catholic Church. In ancient Egypt it was used in rejuvenating face masks, cosmetics, and perfumes. It has been used medicinally in the East and West for a wide range of conditions including syphilis, rheumatism, respiratory and urinary tract infections, skin diseases, as well as digestive and nervous complaints. In addition, frankincense is extensively used in the manufacture of incense, and the gum and oil are used as fragrance components in soaps, cosmetics, and perfumes, especially oriental fragrances.

A pale yellow or greenish mobile liquid with a fresh, terpeney top note and a warm, rich, sweet-balsamic undertone. A handsome small tree or shrub with abundant pinnate leaves and white or pale pink flowers. It yields a natural oleo gum resin.

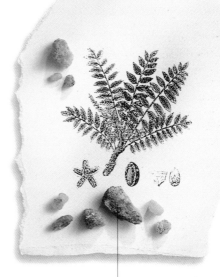

GUM RESIN

DATAFILE

AROMATHERAPY/ HOME USE

Skin Care: *Blemishes, dry and mature complexions, scars, wounds, wrinkles.*

Respiratory System: *Asthma, bronchitis, catarrh, coughs, laryngitis.*

Genitourinary System: *Cystitis, dysmenorrhea, leucorrhea, metrorrhagia.*

Immune System: *Colds, flu.*

Nervous System: *Anxiety, nervous tension, and stress: "Frankincense has, among its physical properties, the ability to slow down and deepen the breath … which is very conducive to prayer and meditation."*[4]

EXTRACTION

Essential oil by steam distillation from oleo gum resin (approx. 3–10 per cent oil to 60–70 per cent resin). An absolute is also produced, used mainly as a fixative.

ACTIONS

Anti-inflammatory, antiseptic, astringent, carminative, cicatrizant, cytophylactic, digestive, diuretic, emmenagogue, expectorant, sedative, tonic, uterine, vulnerary.

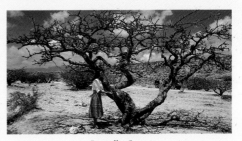

Boswellia Carteri

COMPATIBILITIES

It blends well with sandalwood, pine, vetiver, geranium, lavender, mimosa, orange, bergamot, camphor, basil, pepper, and other spices.

SAFETY DATA
Nontoxic, nonirritant, nonsensitizing

Calamintha

FAMILY: LAMIACEAE (LABIATAE)

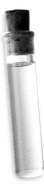

Herbal/Folk Tradition

It has a long history of use as a herbal remedy mainly for nervous and digestive complaints, also menstrual pain, colds, chills, and cramp. Catmint is current in the British Herbal Pharmacopoeia as a specific for flatulent colic in children and for the common cold. Catmint is native to Europe and parts of Asia, and naturalized throughout South Africa and North America, where it is used as a wild cat lure. It is cultivated for its oil throughout the Mediterranean region, former Yugoslavia, Poland and in the USA.

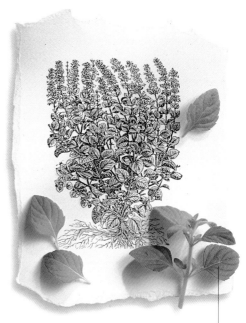

An erect, bushy, perennial plant not more than 3ft (1m) high, with square stems, soft oval serrated leaves grayish-green beneath, and rather inconspicuous pale purple flowers. The whole plant has a strong aromatic scent, which is attractive to cats.

FRESH LEAF

DATAFILE

AROMATHERAPY/ HOME USE

Circulation, Muscles, and Joints:
Chills, cold in the joints, muscular aches and pains, rheumatism.
Digestive System:
Colic, flatulence, nervous dyspepsia.
Nervous System:
Insomnia, nervous tension, and stress-related conditions.

EXTRACTION
Essential oil by steam distillation from the flowering tops.

ACTIONS
Anesthetic (local), antirheumatic, antispasmodic, astringent, carminative, diaphoretic, emmenagogue, febrifuge, nervine, sedative, tonic.

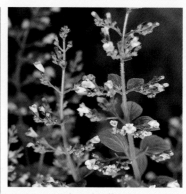

Calamintha officinalis

SAFETY DATA
Nontoxic, nonirritant, nonsensitizing

BURSERA GLABRIFOLIA

Linaloe

FAMILY: BURSERACEAE

Herbal/Folk Tradition

The seed oil is known in India as "Indian lavender oil" and used chiefly as a local perfume ingredient and in soaps by the cosmetics industry of Mysore state. It is not much found outside India.

LINALOE
CHIPPINGS

A tall, bushy tropical shrub or tree, with a smooth bark and bearing fleshy fruit. The wood is used only for distillation purposes when the tree is twenty or thirty years old. The oil is stimulated by lacerating the trunk.

DATAFILE

AROMATHERAPY/ HOME USE
Skin Care: *Acne, cuts, dermatitis, wounds, etc., all skin types.*
Nervous System: *Nervous tension and stress-related conditions.*

EXTRACTION
Essential oil by steam distillation from the wood and seed and husk. (An essential oil is also occasionally produced from the leaves and twigs.)

ACTIONS
Anticonvulsant, anti-inflammatory, antiseptic, bactericidal, deodorant, gentle tonic.

COMPATIBILITIES
It blends well with rose, sandalwood, cedarwood, rosewood, frankincense, floral and woody fragrances.

SAFETY DATA
Nontoxic, nonirritant, nonsensitizing

BULNESIA SARMIENTI

Guaiacwood

FAMILY: ZYGOPHYLLACEAE

Herbal/Folk Tradition

Guaiacwood was once used for treating rheumatism and gout, and is still current in the *British Herbal Pharmacopoeia* as a specific for rheumatism and rheumatoid arthritis.

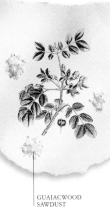

GUAIACWOOD
SAWDUST

A small, wild, tropical tree up to 13ft (4m) high.

DATAFILE

AROMATHERAPY HOME USE
Circulation, Muscles, and Joints: *Arthritis, gout, rheumatoid arthritis.*

EXTRACTION
Essential oil by steam distillation from the broken wood and sawdust. The fluid extract and tincture are used in pharmacology, mainly as a diagnostic reagent in blood texts. Used as a fixative and fragrance component in soaps, cosmetics, and perfumes. Guaiacwood oil is used as a flavor component in most

categories of food product as well as in drinks.

ACTIONS
Anti-inflammatory, antioxidant, antirheumatic, antiseptic, diaphoretic, diuretic, laxative.

COMPATIBILITIES
It blends well with geranium, orange blossom, oakmoss, rose, costus, sandalwood, amyris, spice and woody-floral bases.

SAFETY DATA
Nonirritant, nonsensitizing; possible toxic effects in concentration. Use in moderation. Avoid during pregnancy

CALENDULA OFFICINALIS

Marigold

FAMILY: ASTERACEAE (COMPOSITAE)

Herbal/Folk Tradition

A herb of ancient medical repute, used for skin complaints, menstrual irregularities, varicose veins, hemorrhoids, conjunctivitis, and poor eyesight. The infused oil is used for a wide range of skin problems.

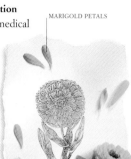

MARIGOLD PETALS

FLOWER HEAD

An annual herb up to 24in (60cm) high with soft, oval, pale green leaves and bright orange, daisylike flowers.

AROMATHERAPY/ HOME USE
The infused oil is very valuable in aromatherapy for its powerful skin-healing properties.

Skin Care: *Burns, cuts, eczema, greasy skin, inflammations, insect bites, rashes, wounds.*

EXTRACTION
An absolute by solvent extraction from the flowers. The real calendula absolute is produced only in small quantities and is difficult to get hold of.

ACTIONS
Antihemorrhagic, anti-inflammatory, antiseptic, antispasmodic, astringent, diaphoretic, cholagogue, cicatrizant, emmenagogue, febrifuge, fungicidal, styptic, tonic, vulnerary.

COMPATIBILITIES
It blends well with oakmoss, hyacinth, floral, and citrus oils.

SAFETY DATA
Nontoxic, nonirritant, nonsensitizing

CANANGA ODORATA VAR. GENUINA

Ylang ylang

FAMILY: ANNONACEAE

Herbal/Folk Tradition

In the Molucca Islands, an ointment is made from ylang ylang and cucuma flowers for cosmetic and hair care, skin diseases, to prevent fever and fight infections.

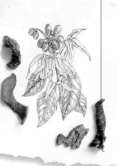

DRIED YLANG YLANG BARK

A tall tropical tree up to 65ft (20m) high with large, tender, fragrant flowers, which can be pink, mauve, or yellow.

AROMATHERAPY/ HOME USE
Skin Care: *Acne, hair growth, hair rinse, insect bites, irritated and oily skin, general skin care.*
Circulation, Muscles, and Joints: *High blood pressure, hypernea, tachycardia, palpitations.*
Nervous System: *Depression, frigidity, impotence, insomnia, nervous tension, and stress. "…soothes and inhibits anger."[5]*

EXTRACTION
Essential oil by water or steam distillation from the freshly picked flowers. The first distillation (about 40 per cent)

is called ylang ylang extra, which is the top grade. An absolute and concrete are also produced by solvent extraction.

ACTIONS
Aphrodisiac, antidepressant, anti-infectious, antiseborrheic, antiseptic, euphoric, hypotensive, nervine, regulator, sedative, stimulant, tonic.

COMPATIBILITIES
It blends well with rosewood, jasmine, vetiver, opopanax, bergamot, mimosa, cassie, Peru balsam, rose, tuberose, and costus,

SAFETY DATA
Nontoxic, nonirritant, possible sensitization especially in those with sensitive skin

CANANGA ODORATA

Cananga

FAMILY: ANNONACEAE

Herbal/Folk Tradition

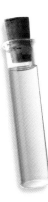

Used locally for infectious illnesses, for example, malaria. The beautiful flowers are also used for decorative purposes at festivals. Cananga is very closely related to the tree that produces ylang ylang oil, but is considered an inferior product in perfumery work; being grown in different regions, the oil has a different quality, being heavier and less delicate than ylang ylang. However, cananga is truly a "complete" oil, whereas ylang ylang is made into several distillates.

Cananga oil is a greenish-yellow or orange viscous liquid with a sweet, floral-balsamic tenacious scent.

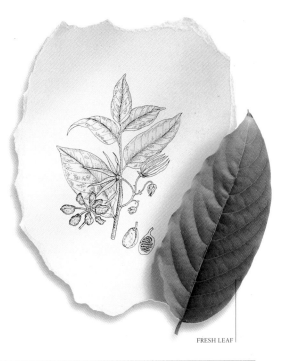

A tall tropical tree, up to 98ft (30m) high, which flowers all year round. It bears large, fragrant, tender, yellow flowers that are virtually identical to those of the ylang ylang.

FRESH LEAF

DATAFILE

AROMATHERAPY/ HOME USE
Skin Care: *Insect bites, fragrance, general skin care.*
Nervous Systems: *Anxiety, depression, nervous tension, and stress-related complaints.*

EXTRACTION
Essential oil by water distillation from the flowers

ACTIONS
Antiseptic, antidepressant, aphrodisiac, hypotensive, nervine, sedative, tonic.

COMPATIBILITIES
It blends well with calamus, birch tar, copaiba balsam, labdanum, orange blossom, oakmoss, jasmine, guaiacwood, and oriental-type bases.

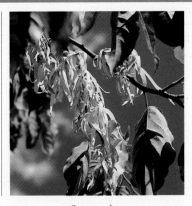

Cananga odorata

SAFETY DATA
Nontoxic, nonirritant, a few cases of sensitization reported. Use in moderation, since its heady scent can cause headaches or nausea

CANARIUM LUZONICUM

Elemi

FAMILY: BURSERACEAE

Herbal/Folk Tradition

The gum or oleoresin is used locally for skin care, respiratory complaints, and as a general stimulant. Elemi was one of the aromatics used by the ancient Egyptians for the embalming process.

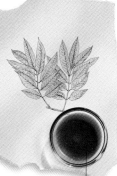

ELEMI RESIN

A tropical tree up to 98ft (30m) high that yields a resinous pathological exudation with a pungent odor. Although it is called a gum, it is almost entirely made up of resin and essential oil.

DATAFILE

AROMATHERAPY/ HOME USE
Skin Care: *Aged skin, infected cuts and wounds, inflammations, rejuvenation, wrinkles – "signifies drying and preservation."[6]*
Respiratory System: *Bronchitis, catarrhal conditions, dry coughs.*
Nervous System: *Nervous exhaustion and stress-related conditions.*

EXTRACTION
Essential oil by steam distillation from the gum. (A resinoid and resin absolute are also produced in small quantities.)

ACTIONS
Antiseptic, balsamic, cicatrizant, expectorant, fortifying, regulatory, stimulant, stomachic, tonic.

COMPATIBILITIES
It blends well with myrrh, frankincense, labdanum, rosemary, lavender, lavandin, sage, cinnamon, and other spices.

SAFETY DATA
Nontoxic, nonirritant, nonsensitizing

CARPHEPHORUS ODORATISSIMUS

Deertongue

FAMILY: ASTERACEAE (COMPOSITAE)

Herbal/Folk Tradition

The roots have been used for their diuretic effects, and applied locally for sore throats and gonorrhea. It is a tonic, used to treat malaria. In folklore it is associated with contraception and sterility in women.

DRIED DEERTONGUE LEAVES

A herbaceous perennial plant distinguished by a naked receptacle and feathery pappus, with large, fleshy, dark green leaves, clasped at the base. The dried leaves have a vanilla-like odor.

DATAFILE

AROMATHERAPY/ HOME USE
None.

EXTRACTION
Oleoresin by solvent extraction from the dried leaves.

ACTIONS
Antiseptic, demulcent, diaphoretic, diuretic, febrifuge, stimulant, tonic.

COMPATIBILITIES
It blends well with oakmoss, labdanum, lavandin, frankincense, clove, patchouli, and oriental-type fragrances.

SAFETY DATA
"Coumarin has toxic properties including liver injury and hemorrhages."[7] Possible dermal irritation and phototoxicity due to the lactones present

CARUM CARVI

Caraway

FAMILY: APIACEAE (UMBELLIFERAE)

Herbal/Folk Tradition

Used extensively as a domestic spice. Traditional remedy for dyspepsia, intestinal colic, menstrual cramps, poor appetite, laryngitis and bronchitis. It promotes milk secretion and is considered specific for flatulent colic in children.

CURVED
CARAWAY
SEEDS

A biennial herb up to 2½ft (75cm) high with a much-branched stem, finely cut leaves, and umbels of white flowers, with a thick and tapering root.

DATAFILE

AROMATHERAPY/ HOME USE
Respiratory System: *Bronchitis, coughs, laryngitis.*
Digestive System: *Dyspepsia, colic, flatulence, gastric spasm, nervous indigestion, poor appetite. See also sweet fennel and dill.*
Immune System: *Colds.*

EXTRACTION
Essential oil by steam distillation from the dried ripe seed or fruit (approximate 2–8 per cent yield).

ACTIONS
Antihistaminic, antimicrobial, antiseptic, aperitif, astringent, carminative, diuretic, emmenagogue, expectorant, galactagogue, larvicidal, stimulant, spasmolytic, stomachic, tonic, vermifuge.

COMPATIBILITIES
It blends well with jasmine, cinnamon, cassia and other spices; however, it is very overpowering.

SAFETY DATA
Nontoxic, nonsensitizing; may cause dermal irritation in concentration

---

CEDRUS ATLANTICA

Atlas cedarwood

FAMILY: PINACEAE

Herbal/Folk Tradition

The oil from the Lebanon cedar was used by the ancient Egyptians for embalming, cosmetics, and perfumery. Traditionally used in the East for bronchial and urinary tract infections, as a preservative, and as an incense.

ATLAS
CEDARWOOD
CONE

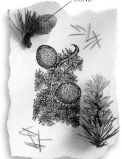

Pyramid-shaped majestic evergreen tree, up to 131ft (40m) high. The wood itself is hard and strongly aromatic because of the high percentage of essential oil it contains.

DATAFILE

AROMATHERAPY/ HOME USE
Skin Care: *Acne, dandruff, dermatitis, eczema, fungal infections, greasy skin, hair loss, skin eruptions, ulcers.*
Circulation, Muscles, and Joints: *Arthritis, rheumatism.*
Respiratory System: *Bronchitis, catarrh, congestion, coughs.*
Genitourinary System: *Cystitis, leucorrhea, pruritis.*
Nervous System: *Nervous tension and stress-related conditions.*

EXTRACTION
Resinoid, absolute, and essential oil by steam distillation from wood, stumps, and sawdust.

ACTIONS
Antiseptic, antiputrescent, antiseborrheic, aphrodisiac, astringent, diuretic, expectorant, fungicidal, mucolytic, sedative (nervous), stimulant (circulatory), tonic.

COMPATIBILITIES
It blends well with rosewood, bergamot, boronia, cypress, calamus, cassie, costus, jasmine, juniper, neroli, mimosa, labdanum, olibanum, clary sage, vetiver, rosemary, ylang ylang, oriental and flower bases.

SAFETY DATA
Nontoxic, nonirritant, nonsensitizing. Best avoided during pregnancy

CHAMAEMELUM NOBILE

Roman chamomile

FAMILY: ASTERACEAE (COMPOSITAE)

Herbal/Folk Tradition

This herb has had a medical reputation in Europe and especially in the Mediterranean region for over 2,000 years, and it is still in widespread use. It was employed by the ancient Egyptians and the Moors, and it was one of the Saxons' nine sacred herbs, which they called "maythen". It was also held to be the "plant's physician", since it promoted the health of plants nearby.

It is current in the *British Herbal Pharmacopoeia* for the treatment of dyspepsia, nausea, anorexia, vomiting in pregnancy, dysmenorrhea, and specifically flatulent dyspepsia associated with mental stress.

A small, stocky, perennial herb, up to 25cm (10in) high, with a much-branched hairy stem, half spreading or creeping. It has feathery pinnate leaves and daisylike white flowers.

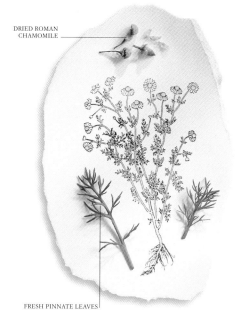

DRIED ROMAN CHAMOMILE

FRESH PINNATE LEAVES

DATAFILE

AROMATHERAPY/ HOME USE

Skin Care: *Acne, allergies, boils, burns, cuts, chilblains, dermatitis, earache, eczema, hair care, inflammations, insect bites, rashes, sensitive skin, teething pain, toothache, wounds.*

Circulation, Muscles, and Joints: *Arthritis, inflamed joints, muscular pain, neuralgia, rheumatism, sprains.*

Digestive System: *Dyspepsia, colic, indigestion, nausea.*

Genitourinary System: *Dysmenorrhea, menopausal problems, menorrhagia.*

Nervous System: *Headache, insomnia, nervous tension,*

migraine, and stress-related complaints.

EXTRACTION

Essential oil by steam distillation of the flowerheads. Used in antiseptic ointments and in carminative, antispasmodic, and tonic preparations. Extensively used in cosmetic, soaps, detergents, high-quality perfumes, and hair and bath products.

ACTIONS

Analgesic, antianemic, antineuralgic, antiphlogistic, antiseptic, antispasmodic, bactericidal, carminative,

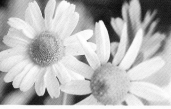

Citrus nobile

cholagogue, cicatrizant, digestive, emmenagogue, febrifuge, hepatic, hypnotic, nerve sedative, stomachic, sudorific, tonic, vermifuge, vulnerary.

COMPATIBILITIES

It blends well with bergamot, clary sage, oakmoss, jasmine, labdanum, orange blossom, rose, geranium, and lavender.

SAFETY DATA

Nontoxic, nonirritant; can cause dermatitis in some individuals

CHENOPODIUM AMBROSIOIDES VAR. ANTHELMINTICUM

Wormseed

FAMILY: CHENOPODIACEAE

Herbal/Folk Tradition

Several Native American
tribes of the eastern
United States use the
whole of the herb
decocted to help ease
painful menstruation
and other female
complaints. It is
also used to expel
roundworm,
hookworm, and
dwarf tapeworm.

DRIED
FLOWERS

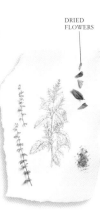

*A hairy, coarse, perennial wayside herb up to 3ft (1m) high
with stout, erect stem, oblong-lanceolate leaves, and many
greenish-yellow flowers, the same color as the leaves.*

DATAFILE

**AROMATHERAPY/
HOME USE**
None. "It should not be used in
therapy, either internally or
externally. and is one of the
most toxic essential oils."⁸
Cases of fatal poisoning have
been reported even in low
doses. Effects can be cumulative.
Due to high ascaridole content,
the oil may explode when
heated or treated with acids.

EXTRACTION
Essential oil by steam distillation
from the whole herb, especially
fruit or seeds.

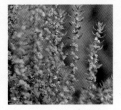

*Chenopodium ambrosioides
var. anthelminticum
Native to South America;
cultivated mainly in east and
southeast United States, also
India, Hungary, and Russia.*

ACTIONS
Anthelmintic, antirheumatic,
antispasmodic, expectorant,
hypotensive.

SAFETY DATA
A very toxic oil

CINNAMOMUM CAMPHORA

Camphor

FAMILY: LAURACEAE

Herbal/Folk Tradition

A long-standing traditional protection against
infectious disease. In addition
it was used for
nervous and
respiratory diseases
in general, and for
heart failure. It is
very poisonous in
large doses.

CAMPHOR BARK

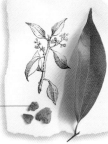

*A tall, handsome, evergreen tree, up to 98ft (30m) high. It
has many branches bearing clusters of small white flowers
followed by red berries. The wood of mature trees produces
a white crystalline substance, the crude camphor.*

DATAFILE

**AROMATHERAPY/
HOME USE**
Brown and yellow camphor
should not be used in therapy.
White camphor may be used
with care for:
Skin Care: *Acne, blemishes,
inflammation, oily conditions; also
for insect prevention.*
Circulation, Muscles, and Joints:
*Arthritis, muscular aches and pains,
rheumatism, sprains, etc.*
Respiratory System: *Bronchitis,
chills, coughs.*
Immune System: *Colds, fever, flu,
infectious diseases.*

EXTRACTION
Crude camphor oil is collected
from trees in crystalline form.
The essential oil is produced by
steam distillation from the wood,
root stumps, and branches and
then rectified under vacuum and
filter pressed to produce three
fractions, known as white, brown,
and yellow camphor.

ACTIONS
Anti-inflammatory, antiseptic,
antiviral, bactericidal, counter-
irritant, diuretic, expectorant,
stimulant, rubefacient, vermifuge.

SAFETY DATA
Brown and yellow camphor (containing safrol) are toxic and carcinogenic. White
camphor does not contain safrol and is relatively nontoxic, nonsensitizing, and
nonirritant. Not compatible with homeopathic treatment

CINNAMOMUM CASSIA

Cassia

FAMILY: LAURACEAE

Herbal/Folk Tradition

Extensively used as a local domestic spice. It is used medicinally mainly for digestive complaints such as flatulent dyspepsia, colic, diarrhea, and nausea, as well as the common cold, rheumatism, and kidney and reproductive complaints.

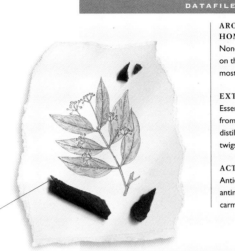

DRIED CASSIA
STALKS

A slender, evergreen tree up to 65ft (20m) high, with leathery leaves and small white flowers. The fruit is approximately the size of a small olive.

DATAFILE

**AROMATHERAPY/
HOME USE**
None. It should never be used on the skin and is one of the most hazardous oils.

EXTRACTION
Essential oil by steam distillation from the leaves, and by water distillation from the bark, leaves, twigs, and stalks.

ACTIONS
Antidiarrheal, antiemetic, antimicrobial, astringent, carminative, spasmolytic.

SAFETY DATA
Dermal toxin, dermal irritant, dermal sensitizer, mucous membrane irritant

CISTUS LADANIFER

Labdanum

FAMILY: CISTACEAE

Herbal/Folk Tradition

One of the early aromatic substances of the ancient world. The gum was used for catarrh, diarrhea, dysentery, and to promote menstruation; externally it was used in plasters.

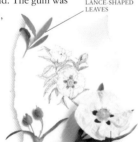

LANCE-SHAPED
LEAVES

FRESH FLOWER

A small sticky shrub up to 10ft (3m) high with lance-shaped leaves that are white and furry on the underside, and fragrant white flowers. Labdanum gum is a natural oleoresin, obtained by boiling the plant material in water.

DATAFILE

**AROMATHERAPY/
HOME USE**
Skin Care: *Mature skin, wrinkles.*
Respiratory System: *Coughs, bronchitis, rhinitis, etc.*
Immune System: *Colds.*

EXTRACTION
A resinoid or resin concrete and absolute by solvent extraction from the crude gum. An essential oil by steam distillation from the crude gum, the absolute, or from the leaves and twigs of the plant.

ACTIONS
Antimicrobial, antiseptic, antitussive, astringent, balsamic, emmenagogue, expectorant, tonic.

COMPATIBILITIES
It blends well with oakmoss, clary sage, pine, juniper, calamus, opopanax, lavender, lavandin, bergamot, cypress, veitiver, sandalwood, patcholi, olibanum, and maroc chamomile.

SAFETY DATA
Generally nontoxic, nonirritant, nonsensitizing. Avoid during pregnancy

CINNAMOMUM ZEYLANICUM

Cinnamon

FAMILY: LAURACEAE

CRUSHED CINNAMON

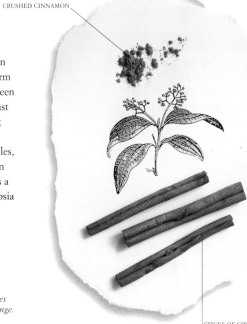

Herbal/Folk Tradition

The inner bark of the new shoots from the cinnamon tree are gathered every two years and used in the form of sticks as a domestic spice. It has been used for thousands of years in the East for a variety of complaints, including colds, flu, digestive and menstrual problems, rheumatism, kidney troubles, and as a general stimulant. Current in the British Herbal Pharmacopoeia as a specific for flatulent colic and dyspepsia with nausea.

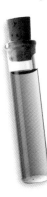

A yellow to brownish liquid with a warm, spicy, somewhat harsh odor.

A tropical evergreen up to 49ft (15m) high, with strong branches and thick scabrous bark with young shoots speckled greeny-orange. It has shiny green leaves, small white flowers, and oval berries.

STICKS OF CINNAMON

DATAFILE

AROMATHERAPY/ HOME USE

Cinnamon bark oil – none. It is one of the most hazardous oils, and should never be used on the skin.
Cinnamon leaf oil:
Skin Care: *Lice, scabies, tooth and gum care, warts, wasp stings.*
Circulation, Muscles, and Joints: *Poor circulation, rheumatism.*
Digestive System: *Anorexia, colitis, diarrhea, dyspepsia, intestinal infection, sluggish digestion, spasm.*
Genitourinary System: *Childbirth (stimulates contractions), frigidity, leucorrhea,* metrorrhagia, scanty periods.
Immune System: *Chills, colds, flu, infectious diseases.*
Nervous System: *Debility, nervous exhaustion, and stress-related conditions.*

EXTRACTION

Essential oil by water or steam distillation from the leaves and twigs, and from the dried inner bark.

ACTIONS

Anthelmintic, antidiarrheal, antidote (to poison), antimicrobial, antiseptic, antispasmodic, antiputrescent, aphrodisiac, astringent, carminative, digestive, emmenagogue, hemostatic, orexigenic, parasiticide, refrigerant, spasmolytic, stimulant (circulatory, cardiac, respiratory), stomachic, vermifuge.

COMPATIBILITIES

It blends well with olibanum, ylang ylang, orange mandarin, benzoin, and Peru balsam.

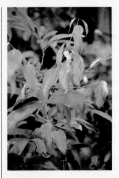

Cinnamon zeylanicum

SAFETY DATA

1. Leaf oil is relatively nontoxic; possibly irritant because of the cinnamaldehyde. Eugenol is irritant to the mucous membranes: use in moderation. 2. Bark oil is a dermal toxin, irritant, and sensitizer; also irritant to the mucous membranes

CITRUS AURANTIFOLIA

Lime

FAMILY: RUTACEAE

Herbal/Folk Tradition

The fruit is often used indiscriminately in place of lemon with which it shares many qualities. It is used for similar purposes including fever, infections, sore throat, colds, etc. In the past was used as a remedy for dyspepsia with glycerin of pepsin.

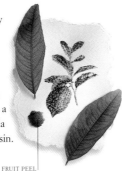

FRUIT PEEL

A small evergreen tree up to 15ft (4.5m) high, with stiff sharp spines, smooth ovate leaves, and small white flowers. The bitter fruit is pale green, about half the size of a lemon.

AROMATHERAPY/ HOME USE

Skin Care: *Acne, anemia, blemishes, brittle nails, boils, chilblains, corns, cuts, greasy skin, herpes, insect bites, mouth ulcers, varicose veins, warts.*

Circulation, Muscles, and Joints: *Arthritis, cellulitis, high blood pressure, nosebleeds, obesity (congestion), poor circulation, rheumatism.*

Respiratory System: *Asthma, throat infections, bronchitis, catarrh.*

Digestive System: *Dyspepsia.*

Immune System: *Colds, flu, fever and infections.*

EXTRACTION

Essential oil by cold expression of the peel of the unripe fruit (preferred in perfumery work) or by steam distillation of the whole ripe crushed fruit (a by-product of the juice industry).

ACTIONS

Antirheumatic, antiscorbutic, antiseptic, antiviral, aperitif, bactericidal, febrifuge, restorative, tonic.

COMPATIBILITIES

It blends well with neroli, citronella, lavender, lavandin, rosemary, clary sage, and other citrus oils.

SAFETY DATA

Nontoxic, nonirritant, nonsensitizing. However, the expressed "peel" oil is phototoxic (but not the steam-distilled "whole fruit" oil)

CITRUS AURANTIUM VAR. AMARA

Bitter orange

FAMILY: RUTACEAE

Herbal/Folk Tradition

The dried bitter orange peel is used as a tonic and carminative in treating dyspepsia. Ingestion of large amounts of orange peel in children, however, is said to cause toxic effects.

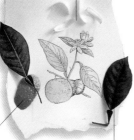

FLOWER PETALS

OUTER PEEL OF FRUIT

FRESH BITTER ORANGE

An evergreen tree up to 33ft (10m) high with dark green, glossy, oval leaves, with long spines. It has a smooth grayish trunk and branches, and fragrant white flowers. The fruits are smaller and darker than the sweet orange.

AROMATHERAPY/ HOME USE

See Sweet Orange page 72.

EXTRACTION

An essential oil by cold expression (hand or machine pressing) from the outer peel of the almost ripe fruit. (A terpeneless oil is also produced.) The leaves are used for the production of petitgrain oil; the blossom for neroli oil.

ACTIONS

Anti-inflammatory, antiseptic, astringent, bactericidal,

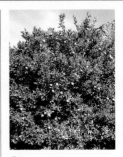

Citrus aurantium var. amara

carminative, choleretic, fungicidal, sedative (mild), stomachic, tonic.

SAFETY DATA

Phototoxic; otherwise generally nontoxic, nonirritant and nonsensitizing. Limonene has been reported to cause contact dermatitis in some individuals

CITRUS AURANTIUM VAR. AMARA

Orange blossom

FAMILY: RUTACEAE

FLOWER PETAL

Herbal/Folk Tradition

This oil, neroli, was named after a princess of Nerola in Italy, who wore it as a perfume. Orange flowers have

many folk associations. They were used in bridal bouquets: to calm nervous apprehension before the couple retired to the marriage bed.

In Europe an infusion of dried flowers is used as a mild stimulant of the nervous system, and as a blood cleanser. The distillation water, known as orange flower water, is a popular cosmetic and household article.

The essential oil is a dark yellow or brownish yellow mobile liquid with a fresh, dry almost floral odor.

An evergreen tree up to 33ft (10m) high with glossy dark green leaves and fragrant white flowers.

ORANGE BLOSSOM LEAVES

DATAFILE

AROMATHERAPY/ HOME USE
Skin Care: *Scars, stretch marks, thread veins, mature and sensitive skin, tones the complexion, wrinkles.*
Circulation, Muscles, and Joints: *Palpitations, poor circulation.*
Digestive system: *Diarrhea (chronic), colic, flatulence, spasm, nervous dyspepsia.*
Nervous system: *Anxiety, depression, nervous tension, PMS, shock, stress-related conditions – "I find that by far the most important uses of neroli are in helping with problems of emotional origin."[9]*

EXTRACTION
A concrete and aboslute are produced by solvent extraction from the freshly picked flowers, and an essential oil is produced by steam distillation. An orange flower water and an absolute are produced as a by-product of the distillation process.

ACTIONS
Antidepressant, antiseptic, antispasmodic, aphrodisiac, bactericidal, carminative, cicatrizant, cordial, deodorant, digestive, fungicidal, hypnotic (mild), stimulant (nervous), tonic (cardiac, circulatory).

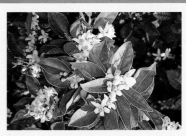

Citrus sinensis

COMPATIBILITIES
It blends well with virtually all oils: chamomile, coriander, geranium, benzoin, clary sage, jasmine, lavender, rose, ylang ylang, lemon, and other citrus oils.

SAFETY DATA
Nontoxic, nonirritant, nonsensitizing, nonphototoxic

CITRUS AURANTIUM VAR. AMARA

Petitgrain

FAMILY: RUTACEAE

Herbal/Folk Tradition

At one time the oil used to be extracted from the green unripe oranges when they were still the size of cherries – hence the name petitgrains or "little grains". One of the classic ingredients of eau-de-cologne.

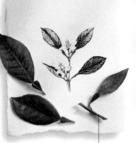

FRESH PETITGRAIN

The oil of petitgrain is produced from the leaves and twigs of the same tree that produces bitter orange oil and orange blossom oil: see Bitter orange, page 68 and Orange blossom, page 69.

DATAFILE

AROMATHERAPY/ HOME USE

Skin Care: *Acne, excessive perspiration, greasy skin and hair, toning.*
Digestive System: *Dyspepsia, flatulence.*
Nervous System: *Convalescence, insomnia, nervous exhaustion, and stress-related conditions.*

EXTRACTION
Essential oil by steam distillation from the leaves and twigs. An orange "leaf and flower" water absolute is also produced, known as *petitgrain sur fleurs.*

ACTIONS
Antiseptic, antispasmodic, deodorant, digestive, nervine, stimulant (digestive, nervous), stomachic, tonic.

COMPATIBILITIES
It blends well with rosemary, lavender, geranium, bergamot, bitter orange, orange blossom, labdanum, oakmoss, clary sage, jasmine, benzoin, palmarosa, clove, and balsams.

SAFETY DATA
Nontoxic, nonirritant, nonsensitizing, nonphototoxic

CITRUS BERGAMIA

Bergamot

FAMILY: RUTACEAE

Herbal/Folk Tradition

Named after the city of Bergamot in Lombardy, where the oil was first sold. The oil has been used in Italy for many years, primarily for worms and fever (including malaria). Also useful for mouth, skin, respiratory, and urinary tract infections.

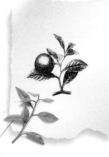

FRESH BERGAMOT

A small tree, about 15ft (4.5m) high with smooth oval leaves, bearing small round fruit that ripen from green to yellow, much like a miniature orange in appearance.

AROMATHERAPY/ HOME USE

Skin Care: *Acne, blemishes, boils, cold sores, eczema, insect repellent and bites, oily skin, psoriasis, scabies, varicose ulcers, wounds.*
Respiratory System: *Halitosis, mouth infections, sore throat.*
Digestive System: *Flatulence, loss of appetite.*
Genitourinary System: *Cystitis, leucorrhea, pruritis, thrush.*
Immune System: *Colds, fever, flu, infectious diseases.*
Nervous System: *Anxiety, depression, and stress.*

EXTRACTION
Essential oil by cold expression of the peel of the fruit.

ACTIONS
Analgesic, anthelmintic, antidepressant, antiseptic (pulmonary, genitourinary), antispasmodic, antitoxic, carminative, digestive, diuretic, deodorant, febrifuge, laxative, parasiticide, rubefacient, stimulant, stomachic, tonic, vermifuge, vulnerary.

SAFETY DATA
Certain furocoumarins, notably bergapten, have been found to be phototoxic in concentration and in dilution even after some time. Extreme care must be taken in dermal applications – or substitute with a rectified or "bergapten-free" oil. Otherwise nontoxic and relatively nonirritant

CITRUS LIMON

Lemon

FAMILY: RUTACEAE

Herbal/Folk Tradition

The juice and peel, high in vitamins A, B, and C, are widely used as a domestic seasoning. It was used for fever, such as malaria and typhoid, and employed for scurvy on English ships. The juice is invaluable for acidic disorders, rheumatism, and dysentery.

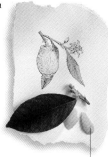

OUTER PEEL OF FRUIT

A small evergreen tree up to 20ft (6m) high with serrated oval leaves, stiff thorns, and very fragrant flowers. The fruit turns from green to yellow on ripening.

DATAFILE	
AROMATHERAPY/ HOME USE See Lime, page 68.	hypotensive, insecticidal, rubefacient, stimulates white corpuscles, tonic, vermifuge.
EXTRACTION Essential oil by cold expression from outer part of fresh peel.	**COMPATIBILITIES** It blends well with citrus oils, lavender, orange blossom, ylang ylang, rose, sandalwood, olibanum, chamomile, benzoin, fennel, geranium, eucalyptus, juniper, oakmoss, lavandin, elemi, labdanum.
ACTIONS Anti-anemic, antimicrobial, antirheumatic, antisclerotic, antiscorbutic, antiseptic, antispasmodic, antitoxic, astringent, bactericidal, carminative, cicatrizant, depurative, diaphoretic, diuretic, febrifuge, hemostatic,	

SAFETY DATA
Nontoxic; may cause dermal irritation or sensitization reactions in some individuals – apply in moderation. Phototoxic – do not use on skin exposed to direct sunlight

CITRUS RETICULATA

Mandarin

FAMILY: RUTACEAE

Herbal/Folk Tradition

In France it is regarded as a safe children's remedy for indigestion, hiccups, etc., and for the elderly since it helps strengthen the digestive function and liver.

OUTER PEEL OF FRUIT

YOUNG MANDARIN SHOOT

CUTTING WITH FLOWER BUDS

A small evergreen tree up to 20ft (6m) high with glossy leaves, fragrant flowers, and bearing fleshy fruit. The tangerine is larger than the mandarin and rounder, with a yellower skin, more like the original Chinese type.

DATAFILE	
AROMATHERAPY/ HOME USE Skin Care: *Acne, blemishes, congested and oily skin, scars, stretch marks, toner.* Circulation, Muscles, and Joints: *Fluid retention, obesity.* Digestive System: *Digestive problems, dyspepsia, hiccoughs, intestinal problems.* Nervous System: *Insomnia, nervous tension, restlessness. It is often used for children and pregnant women and is recommended in synergistic combinations with other citrus oils.*	**EXTRACTION** Essential oil by cold expression from the outer peel. A mandarin petitgrain oil is produced in small quantities by steam distillation from the leaves and twigs. **ACTIONS** Antiseptic, antispasmodic, carminative, digestive, diuretic (mild), laxative (mild), sedative, stimulant (digestive and lymphatic), tonic. **COMPATIBILITIES** It blends well with citrus oils, especially orange blossom, and spice oils such as nutmeg.

SAFETY DATA
Nontoxic, nonirritant, nonsensitizing. Possibly phototoxic, although it has not been demonstrated decisively

CITRUS SINENSIS

Sweet orange

FAMILY: RUTACEAE

Herbal/Folk Tradition

A very nutritious fruit, containing vitamins A, B, and C. In Chinese medicine the dried sweet

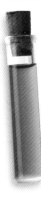

orange peel is used to treat coughs, colds, anorexia, and malignant breast sores. Li Shih-chên says: "The fruits of all the different species and varieties of citrus are considered by the Chinese to be cooling. The sweet varieties increase bronchial secretion and the sour promote expectoration. They all quench thirst, and are stomachic and carminative."[10]

A yellowy-orange or dark orange mobile liquid with a sweet, fresh, fruity scent.

An evergreen tree, smaller than the bitter variety, less hardy with fewer or no spines. The fruit has a sweet pulp and nonbitter membranes.

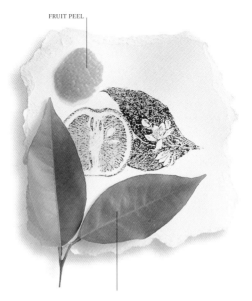

FRUIT PEEL

DATAFILE

AROMATHERAPY/ HOME USE
Skin Care: *Oily skin, mouth ulcers.*
Circulation, Muscles, and Joints: *Obesity, palpitations, water retention.*
Respiratory System: *Bronchitis, chills.*
Digestive System: *Constipation, dyspepsia, spasm.*
Immune System: *Colds, flu.*
Nervous System: *Nervous tension and stress.*

EXTRACTION
Essential oil by cold expression of the fresh ripe or almost ripe outer peel or by steam distillation of the fresh ripe or almost ripe outer peel. An inferior oil is also produced by distillation from the essences recovered as a by-product of orange juice manufacture.

ACTIONS
Antidepressant, anti-inflammatory, antiseptic, bactericidal, carminative, choleretic, digestive, fungicidal, hypotensive, sedative , stimulant (digestive and lymphatic), stomachic, tonic.

COMPATIBILITIES
Lavender, neroli, lemon, clary sage, myrrh, and spice oils, such as nutmeg and cinnamon.

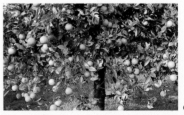

Citrus sinensis

SAFETY DATA

Generally nontoxic (although ingestion of large amounts of orange peel has been known to be fatal to children); distilled orange oil is phototoxic; its use on the skin should be avoided in direct sunlight. There is no evidence that expressed sweet orange oil is phototoxic, nonirritant and nonsensitizing (although limonene has caused dermatitis in a few individuals)

CITRUS X PARADISI

Grapefruit

FAMILY: RUTACEAE

Herbal/Folk Tradition
It shares the nutritional qualities of other citrus species, being high in vitamin C and a valuable protection against infectious illness.

YOUNG FRUIT

FRUIT PEEL

A cultivated tree, often over 33ft (10m) high with glossy leaves and large yellow fruits, believed to have derived from the shaddock (C. grandis).

DATAFILE

AROMATHERAPY/ HOME USE
Skin Care: *Acne, congested and oily skin, promotes hair growth, tones the skin and tissues.*
Circulation, Muscles, and Joints: *Cellulitis, exercise preparation, muscle fatigue, obesity, stiffness, water retention.*
Immune System: *Colds, flu.*
Nervous System: *Depression, headaches, nervous exhaustion, performance stress.*

EXTRACTION
Essential oil by cold expression from the fresh peel.

ACTIONS
Antiseptic, antitoxic, astringent, bactericidal, diuretic, depurative, stimulant (lymphatic, digestive), tonic.

COMPATIBILITIES
It blends well with lemon, palmarosa, bergamot, neroli, rosemary, cypress, lavender, geraniumn, cardomon, and other spice oils.

SAFETY DATA
Nontoxic, nonirritant, nonsensitizing, nonphototoxic.
It has a short shelf life – it oxidizes quickly

COMMIPHORA ERYTHRAEA

Opopanax

FAMILY: BURSERACEAE

Herbal/Folk Tradition
Opopanax, derived from *O. chironium,* has antispasmodic, expectorant, emmenagogue, and antiseptic properties, once used in asthma, hysteria, and visceral afflictions.

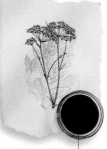

OPOPANAX GUM

A tall tropical tree, similar to myrrh, which contains a natural oleogum resin in tubular vessels between the bark and wood of the trunk. The crude gum dries to form dark reddish-brown tear-shaped lumps.

DATAFILE

AROMATHERAPY/ HOME USE
Possibly similar uses to Myrrh, see page 74.

EXTRACTION
Essential oil by steam (or water) distillation from the crude oleogum resin. A resinoid by solvent extraction from the crude oleogum resin.

ACTIONS
Antiseptic, antispasmodic, balsamic, expectorant.

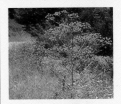

Commiphora erythraea

COMPATIBILITIES
It blends well with clary sage, cilantro, labdanum, bergamot, myrrh, frankincense, vetiver, sandalwood, patchouli, mimosa, fir needle, and neroli.

SAFETY DATA
Frequently adulterated – it is more expensive than the "hirabol myrrh".
The commercial resinoid is also usually mixed with a solvent such as myristate, because it is otherwiseunpourable at room temperatures

COMMIPHORA MYRRHA

Myrrh

FAMILY: BURSERACEAE

CRUDE MYRRH

Herbal/Folk Tradition

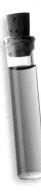

In China it is used for arthritis, menstrual problems, sores, and hemorrhoids. In the West it is considered to have an "opening, heating, drying nature" (Joseph Miller), good for asthma, coughs, common cold, catarrh, sore throat, weak gums and teeth, ulcers, and sores. It has also been used to treat leprosy. Current in the British Herbal Pharmacopoeia as a specific for mouth ulcers, gingivitis, and pharyngitis.

The essential oil is a pale yellow to amber oily liquid with a warm, sweet-balsamic, slightly spicy medicinal odor.

The Commiphora species that yield myrrh are shrubs or small trees up to 33ft (10m) high, with knotted branches, trifolate aromatic leaves, and white flowers.

DATAFILE

AROMATHERAPY/HOME USE

Skin Care: *Athlete's foot, chapped and cracked skin, eczema, mature complexions, ringworm, wounds, wrinkles.*

Circulation, Muscles, and Joints: *Arthritis.*

Respiratory System: *Asthma, bronchitis, catarrh, coughs, gum infections, gingivitis, mouth ulcers, sore throat, voice loss.*

Digestive System: *Diarrhea, dyspepsia, flatulence, hemorrhoids, loss of appetite.*

Genitourinary System: *Amenorrhea, leucorrhea, pruritis, thrush.*

Immune System: *Colds.*

EXTRACTION

Resinoid (and resin absolute) by solvent extraction of the crude myrrh. Essential oil by steam distillation of the crude myrrh.

ACTIONS

Anticatarrhal, anti-inflammatory, antimicrobial, antiphlogistic, antiseptic, astringent, balsamic, carminative, cicatrizant, emmenagogue, expectorant, fungicidal, revitalizing, sedative, stimulant (digestive, pulmonary), stomachic, tonic, uterine, vulnerary.

Myrrh

COMPATIBILITIES

It blends well with frankincense, sandalwood, benzoin, oakmoss, cypress, juniper, mandarin, geranium, patchouli, thyme, mints, lavender, pine, and spices.

SAFETY DATA

Nonirritant, nonsensitizing, possibly toxic in high concentration. Not to be used during pregnancy

COPAIFERA OFFICINALIS

Copaiba balsam

FAMILY: FABACEAE (LEGUMINOSAE)

Herbal/Folk Tradition
Used for centuries in Europe in the treatment of chronic cystitis and bronchitis; also for treating piles, chronic diarrhea, and intestinal problems.

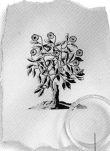

CRUDE COPAIBA BALSAM

Wild-growing tropical tree up to 59ft (18m) high, with thick foliage and many branches. The natural oleoresin occurs as a physiological product from various Copaifera species. Not a "true" balsam.

DATAFILE

AROMATHERAPY/ HOME USE
Digestive System: *Intestinal infections, piles.*
Respiratory System: *Bronchitis, chills, colds, coughs, etc.*
Genitourinary System: *Cystitis.*
Nervous System: *Stress-related conditions.*

EXTRACTION
The crude balsam is collected by drilling holes into the tree trunks. An essential oil is obtained by dry distillation from the crude balsam.

ACTIONS
Bactericidal, balsamic, disinfectant, diuretic, expectorant, stimulant.

COMPATIBILITIES
The crude balsam blends well with styrax, amyris, lavandin, cedarwood, lavender, oakmoss, woods, and spices. The oil blends well with cananga, ylang ylang, vanilla, jasmine, violet, and other florals.

SAFETY DATA
Relatively nontoxic, nonirritant, possible sensitization. Large doses cause vomiting and diarrhea

---

CORIANDRUM SATIVUM

Cilantro

FAMILY: APIACEAE (UMBELLIFERAE)

Herbal/Folk Tradition
The seeds and leaves are widely used as a garnish and domestic spice. It has also been used in the form of an infusion for children's diarrhea, digestive upsets, griping pains, anorexia, and flatulence.

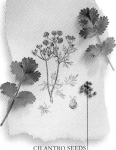

CILANTRO SEEDS

An aromatic annual herb about 3ft (1m) high with bright green delicate leaves, umbels of lacelike white flowers, followed by a mass of green (turning brown) round seeds.

DATAFILE

AROMATHERAPY/ HOME USE
Circulation, Muscles, and Joints: *Accumulated fluids and toxins, arthritis, gout, muscular aches and pains, poor circulation, rheumatism, stiffness.*
Digestive System: *Anorexia, colic, diarrhea, dyspepsia, flatulence, nausea, piles, spasm.*
Immune System: *Colds, flu, infections (general), measles.*
Nervous System: *Debility, migraine, neuralgia, exhaustion.*

EXTRACTION
Essential oil by steam distillation from the crushed ripe seeds.

ACTIONS
Analgesic, aperitif, aphrodisiac, antioxidant, antirheumatic, antispasmodic, bactericidal, depurative, digestive, carminative, cytotoxic, fungicidal, larvicidal, lipolytic, revitalizing, stimulant (cardiac, circulatory, nervous system), stomachic.

COMPATIBILITIES
It blends well with clary sage, bergamot, jasmine, olibanum, neroli, petitgrain, citronella, sandalwood, cypress, pine, ginger, cinnamon, and other spice oils.

SAFETY DATA
Generally nontoxic, nonirritant, nonsensitizing. Stupefying in large doses – use in moderation

CROTON ELEUTERIA

Cascarilla bark

FAMILY: EUPHORBIACEAE

Herbal/Folk Tradition

The bark is used as an aromatic bitter and tonic for dyspepsia, diarrhea, dysentery, fever, debility, nausea, flatulence, vomiting, and chronic bronchitis. The leaves are used as a digestive tea and to flavor tobacco.

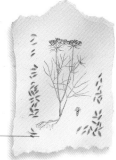

CASCARILLA BARK

A large shrub or small tree up to 39ft (12m) high, with ovate silver-bronze leaves, pale yellowish-brown bark, and small white fragrant flowers. It bears fruits and flowers all year round.

DATAFILE

AROMATHERAPY/ HOME USE
Respiratory System: *Bronchitis, coughs.*
Digestive System: *Dyspepsia, flatulence, nausea.*
Immune System: *Flu.*

EXTRACTION
Essential oil by steam distillation from the dried bark (1.5–3 per cent yield).

ACTIONS
Astringent, antimicrobial, antiseptic, carminative, digestive, expectorant, stomachic, tonic.

COMPATIBILITIES
It blends well with nutmeg, pepper, pimento, sage, oakmoss, oriental and spicy bases.

SAFETY DATA
Nonirritant, nonsensitizing, relatively nontoxic (possibly narcotic in large doses)

CUMINUM CYMINUM

Cumin

FAMILY: APIACEAE (UMBELLIFERAE)

Herbal/Folk Tradition

A traditional Middle Eastern spice, and one of the main ingredients of curry. It is used in Ayurvedic medicine as a stimulant, especially for digestive problems such as colic, sluggish digestion, and dyspepsia.

CUMIN SEED

A small, delicate, annual herb about 20in (50cm) high with a slender stem, dark green feathery leaves, and small pink or white flowers followed by small oblong seeds.

DATAFILE

AROMATHERAPY/ HOME USE
Circulation, Muscles, and Joints: *Accumulation of fluids or toxins, poor circulation.*
Digestive System: *Colic, dyspepsia, flatulence, indigestion, spasm.*
Nervous System: *Debility, headaches, migraine, nervous exhaustion.*

EXTRACTION
Essential oil by steam distillation from the ripe seeds.

ACTIONS
Antioxidant, antiseptic, antispasmodic, antitoxic, aphrodisiac, bactericidal, carminative, depurative, digestive, diuretic, emmenagogue, larvicidal, nervine, stimulant, tonic.

COMPATIBILITIES
It blends well with lavender, lavandin, rosemary, galbanum, rosewood, cardomon, and oriental-type fragrances.

SAFETY DATA
Generally nontoxic, nonirritant, and nonsensitizing; however, the oil is phototoxic – do not expose treated skin to direct sunlight. Avoid during pregnancy

CUPRESSUS SEMPERVIRENS

Cypress

FAMILY: CUPRESSACEAE

Herbal/Folk Tradition

Highly valued as a medicine and as an incense by ancient civilizations, it benefits the urinary system and is considered useful where there is excessive loss of fluid, such as heavy perspiration or menstrual loss and diarrhea.

FRESH CYPRESS

A tall evergreen tree with slender branches and a statuesque conical shape. It bears small flowers and round, brownish-gray cones or nuts.

DATAFILE	
AROMATHERAPY/ HOME USE	**EXTRACTION**
Skin Care: *Hemorrhoids, oily and overhydrated skin, excessive perspiration, insect repellent, pyorrhea (bleeding gums), varicose veins, wounds.*	Essential oil by steam distillation from the needles, twigs, and, occasionally, cones.
Circulation, Muscles, and Joints: *Cellulitis, muscular cramp, edema, poor circulation, rheumatism.*	**ACTIONS** Antirheumatic, antiseptic, antispasmodic, astringent, deodorant, diuretic, hepatic, styptic, sudorific, tonic, vasoconstrictive.
Respiratory System: *Asthma, bronchitis, coughing spasms.*	
Genitourinary System: *Dysmenorrhea, menopausal problems, menorrhagia.*	**COMPATIBILITIES** Cedarwood, pine, lavender, mandarin, clary sage, lemon, cardomon, juniper, Moroccan chamomile, orange ambrette seed, labdanum, benzoin, bergamot, and marjoram.
Nervous System: *Nervous tension and stress.*	

SAFETY DATA
Nontoxic, nonirritant, and nonsensitizing

CURCUMA LONGA

Turmeric

FAMILY: ZINGIBERACEAE

Herbal/Folk Tradition

A common spice, especially for curry powder. It is high in minerals and vitamins, especially vitamin C. It is widely used as a local home remedy. It was once used as a cure for jaundice.

TURMERIC ROOT

A perennial tropical herb up to 3ft (1m) high, with a thick rhizome root, deep orange inside, lanceolate root leaves tapering at each end, and dull yellow flowers.

DATAFILE	
AROMATHERAPY/ HOME USE	
Circulation, Muscles, and Joints: *Arthritis, muscular aches and pains, rheumatism.*	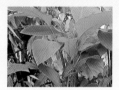
Digestive System: *Anorexia, sluggish digestion, liver congestion.*	*Curcuma longa*
EXTRACTION Essential oil by steam distillation from the "cured" rhizome. An oleoresin, absolute, and concrete are made by solvent extraction.	bactericidal, cholagogue, digestive, diuretic, hypotensive, insecticidal, laxative, rubefacient, stimulant.
ACTIONS Analgesic, antiarthritic, anti-inflammatory, antioxidant,	**COMPATIBILITIES** Cananga, labdanum, elecampane, ginger, orris, cassie, clary sage, and mimosa.

SAFETY DATA
The ketone "tumerone" is moderately toxic and irritant in high concentration. Possible sensitization problems

CYMBOPOGON CITRATUS

Lemongrass

FAMILY: POACEAE (GRAMINEAE)

Herbal/Folk Tradition

Employed in traditional Indian medicine for infectious illness and fever; modern research carried out in India shows that it also acts as a sedative on the central nervous system. It is also used as an insecticide and for food flavoring.

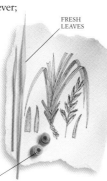

FRESH LEAVES

SLICED LEMONGRASS STEM

A fast-growing, tall, aromatic perennial grass up to 5ft (1.5m) high, producing a network of roots and rootlets that rapidly exhaust the soil.

CYMBOPOGON MARTINII VAR. MARTINII

Palmarosa

FAMILY: GRAMINACEAE

Herbal/Folk Tradition

Formerly knwon as "Indian" or "Turkish" geranium oil, a term that dates back to the time when the oil was shipped from Bombay to the Red Sea and on to Constantinople and Bulgaria, where the oil was often used to adulterate rose oil.

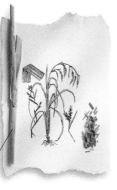

DRIED PALMAROSA STEM

A wild-growing herbaceous plant with long slender stems with terminal flowering tops and fragrant grassy leaves.

CYMBOPOGON NARDUS

Citronella

FAMILY: POACEAE (GRAMINEAE)

Herbal/Folk Tradition

The leaves of citronella are used for their aromatic and medicinal value in many cultures, for fever, intestinal parasites, digestive and menstrual problems, as a stimulant, and an insect repellent. It is used in Chinese traditional medicine for rheumatic pain.

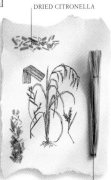

DRIED CITRONELLA

FRESH CITRONELLA GRASS

A tall, aromatic, perennial grass, which has derived from the wild-growing "managrass" found in Sri Lanka.

DATAFILE

AROMATHERAPY/ HOME USE

Skin Care: *Excessive perspiration, oily skin, insect repellent. Mixed with cedarwood oil Virginia, it was a popular remedy against mosquito attacks before the advent of DDT and modern insecticides.*

Immune System: *Cold, flu, minor infections.*

Nervous System: *Fatigue, headaches, migraine, neuralgia.*

EXTRACTION

Essential oil by steam distillation of the fresh, part-dried, or dried grass.

ACTIONS

Antiseptic, antispasmodic, bactericidal, deodorant, diaphoretic, diuretic, emmenagogue, febrifuge, fungicidal, insecticide, stomachic, tonic, vermifuge.

COMPATIBILITIES

It blends well with geranium, lemon, bergamot, orange, cedarwood, and pine.

SAFETY DATA

Nontoxic, nonirritant; may cause dermatitis in some individuals. Avoid during pregnancy

---

DAUCUS CAROTA

Carrot seed

FAMILY: APIACEAE (UMBELLIFERAE)

Herbal/Folk Tradition

A highly nutritious plant, containing substantial amounts of vitamins A, C, B1, and B2. The seeds are used for treating the retention of urine, colic, kidney and digestive disorders, and to promote menstruation.

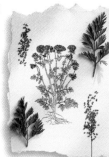

CARROT FRUIT (SEED)

Annual or biennial herb with a 5-ft (1.5-m) high branched stem with hairy leaves and umbels of white lacy flowers.

DATAFILE

AROMATHERAPY/ HOME USE

Skin Care: *Dermatitis, eczema, psoriasis, rashes, revitalize, toning, mature complexions, wrinkles.*

Circulation, Muscles, and Joints: *Toxin accumulation, arthritis, gout, edema, rheumatism.*

Digestive System: *Anemia, anorexia, colic, indigestion, liver congestion.*

Genitourinary and Endocrine Systems: *Amenorrhea, dysmenorrhea, glandular problems, PMS.*

EXTRACTION

Essential oil by steam distillation from the dried fruit.

ACTIONS

Anthelmintic, antiseptic, carminative, depurative, diuretic, emmenagogue, hepatic, stimulant, tonic, vasodilatory, and smooth muscle relaxant.

COMPATIBILITIES

It blends well with costus, cassie, mimosa, cedarwood, geranium, citrus and spice oils.

SAFETY DATA

Nontoxic, nonirritant, nonsensitizing

DIPTERYX ODORATA

Tonka

FAMILY: LEGUMINOSAE

Herbal/Folk Tradition
In the Netherlands the fatty
substance from the beans is sold
as "taquin butter", which used to
be used as an insecticide against
moths in linen closets. The fluid
extract has also been used in
cases of whooping cough.

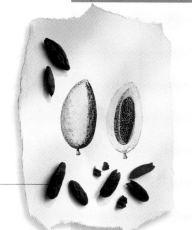

TONKA BEANS

*A very large tropical tree with big elliptical leaves and violet
flowers, bearing fruit that contain a single black seed or
"tonka bean," about the size of a lima bean. The beans are
collected and dried and soaked in alcohol or rum to make
them swell.*

DATAFILE

**AROMATHERAPY/
HOME USE**
None.

EXTRACTION
A concrete and absolute by
solvent extraction from the
"cured" beans.

ACTIONS
Insecticidal, narcotic, tonic
(cardiac).

COMPATIBILITIES
It blends well with lavender,
lavandin, clary sage, styrax,
bergamot, oakmoss,
helichrysum, and citronella.

SAFETY DATA
Oral and dermal toxin, due to high coumarin content

ELETTARIA CARDAMOMUM

Cardomon

FAMILY: ZINGIBERACEAE

Herbal/Folk Tradition
Used extensively as a domestic spice.
It has been used in traditional
Chinese and Indian
medicine for over
3,000 years,
especially for
pulmonary disease,
fever, digestive and
urinary complaints.

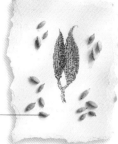

CARDOMON SEEDS

*A perennial, reedlike herb up to 13ft (4m) high, with long,
silk blade-shaped leaves. Its long sheathing stems bear small
yellowish flowers with purple tips, followed by oblong red-
brown seeds.*

DATAFILE

**AROMATHERAPY/
HOME USE**
Digestive System: *Anorexia, colic,
cramp, dyspepsia, flatulence,
griping pains, halitosis, heartburn,
indigestion, vomiting.*
Nervous System: *Mental fatigue,
nervous strain.*

EXTRACTION
Essential oil by steam distillation
from the dried ripe fruit
(seeds). An oleoresin is also
produced in small quantities.

ACTIONS
Antiseptic, antispasmodic,
aphrodisiac, carminative,
cephalic, digestive, diuretic,
sialagogue, stimulant, stomachic,
tonic (nerve).

COMPATIBILITIES
It blends well with rose,
olibanum, orange, bergamot,
cinnamon, cloves, caraway,
ylang ylang, labdanum,
cedarwood, orange blossom,
and oriental bases in general.

SAFETY DATA
Nontoxic, nonirritant, nonsensitizing

DRYOBALANOPS AROMATICA

Borneol

FAMILY: DIPTEROCARPACEAE

Herbal/Folk Tradition

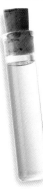

Borneol has long been regarded as a panacea by many
Eastern civilizations, especially in ancient Persia, India, and
China. It was used as a powerful remedy against
plague and other infectious diseases, stomach
and bowel complaints. In China it was also used
for embalming purposes. "It is mentioned by
Marco Polo in the thirteenth century and
Camoens in 1571 who called it the 'balsam of
disease.'"[11] It is valued for ceremonial purposes
in the East generally, and in China particularly
for funeral rites. Its odor repels insects and ants,
and it is therefore highly regarded as lumber for
the construction of buildings.

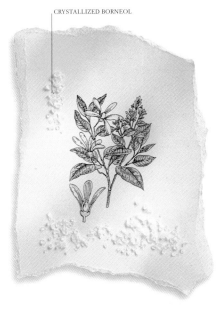

CRYSTALLIZED BORNEOL

*The camphora tree grows to a great height, a majestic tree often
over 82ft (25m) high, with a thick trunk up to 6ft (2m) in diameter.
Borneol is a natural exudation found beneath the bark in crevices
and fissures of some mature trees (about 1 per cent); young trees
produce only a clear yellow liquid known as "liquid camphor".*

DATAFILE

**AROMATHERAPY
HOME USE**

Skin Care: *Cuts, bruises, insect
repellent.*

Circulation, Muscles, and Joints:
*Debility, poor circulation,
rheumatism, sprains.*

Respiratory System: *Bronchitis,
coughs.*

Immune System: *Colds, fever, flu,
and other infectious diseases.*

Nervous System: *Nervous
exhaustion, stress-related
conditions, neuralgia.*

EXTRACTION
The borneol is collected from
the tree trunk in its crude
crystalline form (the locals test
each tree first by making
incisions in the trunk to detect
its presence). The so-called oil
of borneol is extracted by
steam distillation of the wood.

ACTIONS
Mildly analgesic, antidepressant,
antiseptic, antispasmodic,
antiviral, carminative,
rubefacient, stimulant of the
adrenal cortex, tonic (cardiac
and general).

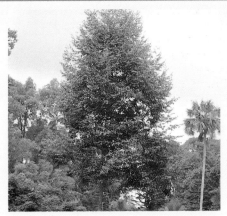

Dryobalanops aromatica

SAFETY DATA
Nontoxic, nonsensitizing, dermal irritant in concentration

Lemon-scented eucalyptus

FAMILY: MYRTACEAE

Herbal/Folk Tradition

Used traditionally for perfuming the linen closet by enclosing the dried leaves in a small sachet. During the last century it was seen as a good insect repellent, especially for cockroaches and silverfish.

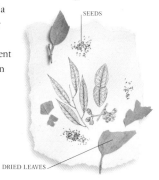

SEEDS

DRIED LEAVES

A tall evergreen tree with a smooth dimpled bark, blotched in gray, cream, and pink. The young leaves are oval, the mature leaves narrow and tapering.

DATAFILE

AROMATHERAPY/ HOME USE
Not compatible with homeopathic treatment.
Skin Care: *Athlete's foot and other fungal infections (e.g. candida), cuts, dandruff, herpes, insect repellent, scabs, sores, wounds.*
Respiratory System: *Asthma, laryngitis, sore throat.*
Immune System: *Colds, fevers, infectious skin conditions such as chickenpox, infectious disease.*

EXTRACTION
Essential oil by steam distillation from the leaves and twigs.

ACTIONS
Antiseptic, antiviral, bactericidal, deodorant, expectorant, fungicidal, insecticide.

SAFETY DATA
Nontoxic, nonirritant, possible sensitization in some individuals. Eucalyptus oil is toxic when taken internally – see blue gum eucalyptus.

Broad-leaved peppermint eucalyptus

FAMILY: MYRTACEAE

Herbal/Folk Tradition

The Aborigines used the burning leaves in the form of a fumigation for the relief of fever: "heat went out of sick man and into fire."

SEEDS

DRIED LEAVES

A robust, medium-size eucalyptus tree, with a short trunk, spreading branches and fibrous gray bark. The young leaves are blue and heart-shaped, the mature leaves are very aromatic, thick, and tapering at both ends.

DATAFILE

AROMATHERAPY/ HOME USE
Not compatible with homeopathic treatment.
Skin Care: *Cuts, sores, ulcers, etc.*
Circulation, Muscles, and Joints: *Arthritis, muscular aches and pains, rheumatism, sports injuries, sprains,*
Respiratory System: *Asthma, bronchitis, catarrh, coughs, throat and mouth infection.*
Immune System: *Colds, fevers, flu, infectious illnesses, e.g. measles.*
Nervous System: *Headaches, nervous exhaustion, neuralgia, sciatica.*

EXTRACTION
Essential oil by steam distillation from the leaves and twigs.

ACTIONS
Analgesic, antineuralgic, antirheumatic, antiseptic, antispasmodic, antiviral, balsamic, cicatrizant, decongestant, deodorant, depurative, diuretic, expectorant, febrifuge, hypoglycemic, parasiticide, prophylactic, rubefacient, stimulant, vermifuge, vulnerary.

SAFETY DATA
Nontoxic, nonirritant (in dilution), nonsensitizing. Eucalyptus oil is toxic if taken internally, see blue gum eucalyptus page 83

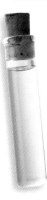

EUCALYPTUS GLOBULUS VAR. GLOBULUS

Blue gum eucalyptus

FAMILY: MYRTACEAE *LAVANDULA ANGUSTIFOLIA*

Herbal/Folk Tradition

A traditional household remedy in Australia, the leaves and oil are used especially for respiratory ailments such as bronchitis and croup, and the dried leaves are smoked like tobacco for asthma. It is also used for feverish conditions (malaria, typhoid, cholera, etc.) and skin problems such as burns, ulcers, and wounds. Aqueous extracts are used for aching joints, bacterial dysentery, ringworms, tuberculosis, etc. and employed for similar reasons in Western and Eastern medicine. The wood is also used for lumber production in Spain.

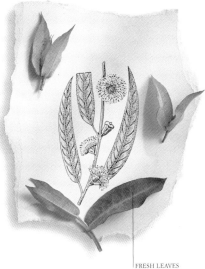

A beautiful, tall, evergreen tree, up to 295ft (90m) high. The young trees have bluish-green oval leaves while the mature trees develop long, narrow, yellowish leaves, creamy-white flowers, and a smooth, pale gray bark often covered with a white powder.

FRESH LEAVES

DATAFILE

AROMATHERAPY/ HOME USE

Not compatible with homeopathic treatment.

Skin Care: *Burns, blisters, cuts, herpes, insect bites, insect repellent, lice, skin infections, wounds.*

Circulation, Muscles, and Joints: *Muscular aches and pains, poor circulation, rheumatoid arthritis, sprains, etc.*

Respiratory System: *Asthma, bronchitis, catarrh, coughs, sinusitis, throat infections.*

Genitourinary System: *Cystitis, leucorrhea.*

Immune System: *Chickenpox, colds, epidemics, flu, measles.*

Nervous System: *Debility, headaches, neuralgia.*

EXTRACTION

Essential oil by steam distillation from the fresh or partially dried leaves and young twigs.

ACTIONS

See Broad-leaved peppermint eucalyptus, page 82.

COMPATIBILITIES

It blends well with thyme, rosemary, lavender, marjoram, pine, cedarwood, and lemon.

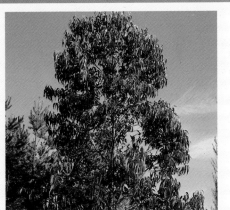

Eucalyptus globulus var. globulus

SAFETY DATA

Externally nontoxic, nonirritant (in dilution), nonsensitizing. "When taken internally eucalyptus oil is toxic and as little as 3.5ml has been reported as fatal."[12]

EVERNIA PRUNASTRI

Oakmoss

FAMILY: USNEACEAE

Herbal/Folk Tradition

Sticta pulmonaceae, a greeny-brown lichen frequently harvested along with *E. prunastri*, is also called oak lungs, lung moss, lungwort, or "lungs of oak" by the Native Americans who use it for respiratory complaints and for treating wounds.

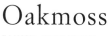

OAK BARK

OAKMOSS LICHEN

A light green lichen found growing primarily on oak trees, sometimes on other species.

DATAFILE	
AROMATHERAPY/ HOME USE As a fixative.	**ACTIONS** Antiseptic, demulcent, expectorant, fixative.
EXTRACTION A range of products is produced: a concrete and an absolute by solvent extraction from the lichen that has often been soaked in lukewarm water prior to extraction; an absolute oil by vacuum distillation of the concrete; resins and resinoids by alcohol extraction of the raw material. Most important of these products is the absolute.	**COMPATIBILITIES** The concrete, resin, and resinoids have a high fixative value and blend with virtually all other oils: they are extensively used in perfumery to lend body and rich natural undertones to all perfume types.

SAFETY DATA
Extensively compounded or bouqueted by cutting or adulteration with other lichen or synthetic perfume materials

FERULA ASSA-FOETIDA

Asafetida

FAMILY: APIACEAE (UMBELLIFERAE)

Herbal/Folk Tradition

Reputed to treat various ailments including asthma, bronchitis, coughs, convulsions, constipation, flatulence, and hysteria. In Chinese medicine it is used to treat neurasthenia.

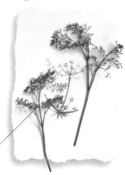

FRESH ASAFETIDA

A large branching perennial herb up to 10ft (3m) high, with a thick fleshy root system and pale yellow-green flowers.

DATAFILE	
AROMATHERAPY/ HOME USE Respiratory System: *"There is evidence that the volatile oil is expelled through the lungs, therefore it is excellent for asthma, bronchitis, whooping cough, etc."[13]* Nervous System: *Fatigue, nervous exhaustion, and stress-related conditions.*	**EXTRACTION** The oleoresin is obtained by making incisions into the root and plant. The juice leaks and harden into dark reddish lumps, before being collected. The essential oil is obtained from the resin by steam distillation. **ACTIONS** Antispasmodic, carminative, expectorant, hypotensive, stimulant.

SAFETY DATA
Available information indicates the oil to be relatively nontoxic and nonirritant. However, it has the reputation for being the most adulterated "drug" on the market. Before being sold, the oleoresin is often mixed with red clay or similar substitutes

FERULA GALBANIFLUA

Galbanum

FAMILY: APIACEAE (UMBELLIFERAE)

Herbal/Folk Tradition

It was used by the ancient civilizations as an incense, and in Egypt for cosmetics and in the embalming process. It is generally used in the East in a similar way to asafetida: for treating wounds, inflammations, and skin disorders and also for respiratory, digestive, and nervous complaints. Zalou root (*F. hermonic*) is used in Beirut as an aphrodisiac.

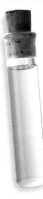

A colorless, or pale yellow or olive liquid with a fresh green top note and woody-dry balsamic undertone.

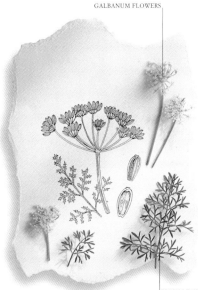

GALBANUM FLOWERS

FRESH LEAVES

A large perennial herb with a smooth stem, shiny leaflets, and small flowers. It contains resin ducts that exude a milky juice, a natural oleoresin. The dried resinous exudation is collected by making incisions at the base of the stem.

DATAFILE

AROMATHERAPY/ HOME USE

Skin Care: *Abscesses, acne, boils, cuts, heals scar tissue, inflammations, tones the skin, mature skin, wrinkles, wounds –* "signifies drying and preservation."[14]

Circulation, Muscles, and Joints: *Poor circulation, muscular aches and pains, rheumatism.*

Respiratory System: *Asthma, bronchitis, catarrh, chronic coughs.*

Digestive System: *Cramp, flatulence, indigestion.*

Nervous System: *Nervous tension and stress-related complaints.*

EXTRACTION

Essential oil by water or steam distillation from the oleoresin or gum – only the Levant or soft type is used for oil production. A partially deterpenized oil is produced, known as "galbanol".

ACTIONS

Analgesic, anti-inflammatory, antimicrobial, antiseptic, antispasmodic, aphrodisiac, balsamic, carminative, cicatrizant, digestive, diuretic, emmenagogue, expectorant, hypotensive, restorative, tonic.

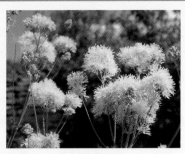

Ferula galbaniflua

COMPATIBILITIES

Hyacinth, violet, narcissus, lavender, geranium, oakmoss, opopanax, pine, fir, styrax, and oriental bases.

SAFETY DATA
Nontoxic, nonirritant, nonsensitizing

FOENICULUM VULGARE

Fennel

FAMILY: APIACEAE (UMBELLIFERAE)

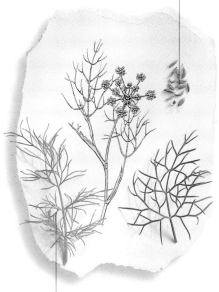

FENNEL SEEDS

Herbal/Folk Tradition

A herb of ancient medical repute, believed to convey longevity, courage, and strength. It was also used to

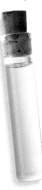

ward off evil spirits, strengthen the eyesight, and neutralize poisons. It is considered good for obstructions of the liver, spleen, and gall bladder and for digestive complaints. It has traditionally been used for obesity, which may be due to a type of estrogenic action, which also increases the milk of nursing mothers. Still current in the British Herbal Pharmacopoeia, used locally for conjunctivitis, blepharitis, and pharyngitis.

Biennial or perennial herb up to 6ft (2m) high, with feathery leaves and golden yellow flowers. There are two main varieties of fennel: bitter or common fennel, slightly taller with less divided leaves occurring in a cultivated or wild form; and sweet fennel (also known as Roman, garden, or French fennel), which is always cultivated.

FRESH FENNEL LEAVES

DATAFILE

AROMATHERAPY/ HOME USE
Bitter fennel: *none.*
Sweet fennel:
Skin Care: *Bruises, dull, oily, mature complexions, pyorrhea.*
Circulation, Muscles, and Joints: *Cellulitis, obesity, edema, rheumatism.*
Respiratory System: *Asthma, bronchitis.*
Digestive System: *Anorexia, colic, constipation, dyspepsia, flatulence, hiccough, nausea.*
Genitourinary System: *Amenorrhea, insufficient milk (in nursing mothers), menopausal problems.*

EXTRACTION
Essential oil by steam distillation. Sweet fennel oil is made from crushed seeds, and bitter fennel oil from crushed seeds or the whole herb (the wild "weed").

ACTIONS
Aperitif, anti-inflammatory, antimicrobial, antiseptic, antispasmodic, carminative, depurative, diuretic, emmenagogue, expectorant, galactagogue, laxative, orexigenic, stimulant (circulatory), splenic, stomachic, tonic, vermifuge.

Foeniculum vulgare

COMPATIBILITIES
Sweet fennel oil blends well with geranium, lavender, rose, and sandalwood.

SAFETY DATA

Nonirritant, relatively nontoxic, narcotic in large doses; bitter fennel may cause sensitization. Bitter fennel oil should not be used on the skin at all, although it is considered superior medicinally. Neither oil should be used by epileptics or during pregnancy. Use in moderation

GARDENIA JASMINOIDES

Gardenia

FAMILY: RUBIACEAE

Herbal/Folk Tradition

The flowers are used locally to flavor tea, much like jasmine.

DRIED GARDENIA BUDS

A decorative bush, often grown for ornamental purposes, bearing fragrant white flowers.

AROMATHERAPY/ HOME USE
Perfume.

EXTRACTION
An absolute (and concrete) by solvent extraction from the fresh flowers.

ACTIONS
Antiseptic, aphrodisiac.

COMPATIBILITIES
It blends well with ylang ylang, jasmine, tuberose, orange blossom, rose, spice and citrus oils

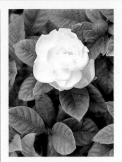

Gardenia jasminoides Native to the Far East, India, and China. Efforts to produce the oil commercially have been largely unsuccessful.

SAFETY DATA
Safety data unavailable at present. Almost all gardenia oil is now synthetically produced

---

GAULTHERIA PROCUMBENS

Wintergreen

FAMILY: ERICACEAE

Herbal/Folk Tradition

The plant has been used for respiratory conditions such as chronic mucus discharge, but is employed mainly for joint and muscular problems such as lumbago, sciatica, neuralgia.

FRESH WINTERGREEN

A small evergreen herb up to 6in (15cm) high with slender creeping stems shooting forth erect twigs with leathery serrated leaves and drooping white flowers, which are followed by fleshy scarlet berries.

AROMATHERAPY/ HOME USE
None. Avoid use, both internally and externally.

EXTRACTION
Essential oil by steam (or water) distillation from the leaf, previously macerated in warm water.

ACTIONS
Analgestic (mild), anti-inflammatory, antirheumatic, antitussive, astringent, carminative, diuretic, emmenagogue, galactagogue, stimulant.

COMPATIBILITIES
It blends well with oregano, mints, thyme, ylang ylang, narcissus, and vanilla.

SAFETY DATA
Toxic, irritant, and sensitizing – an environmental hazard or marine pollutant. The true oil is almost obsolete, having been replaced by synthetic methyl salicylate. See also Sweet birch oil, page 55

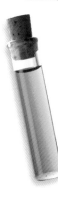

HUMULUS LUPULUS

HUMULUS LUPULUS

Hops
FAMILY: MORACEAE

Herbal/Folk Tradition

Best known as a nerve remedy, for insomnia, nervous tension, neuralgia, and also for sexual neurosis in both sexes. It supports the female estrogens and is useful for amenorrhea (absence of periods). It also acts as a mild sedative, commonly used in the form of the hop pillow where the heavy aromatic odor has been shown to relax by direct action at the olfactory centers. It has also been used for heart disease, and stomach and liver complaints, including bacterial dysentery.

In China it is used for pulmonary tuberculosis and cystitis. It is used to make beer. Current in the British Herbal Pharmacopoeia as a specific for restlessness with nervous headaches and/or indigestion.

Perennial creeping, twining herb up to 26ft (8m) high, which bears male and female flowers on separate plants. It has dark green, heart-shaped leaves and greeny-yellow flowers. A volatile oil, called lupulin, is formed in the glandular hairs of the cones or "strobiles".

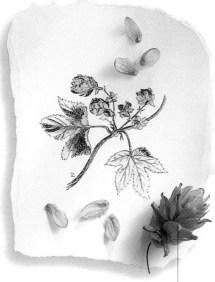

DRIED HOPS

DATAFILE

AROMATHERAPY/ HOME USE

Skin Care: *Dermatitis, rashes, rough skin, ulcers.*

Respiratory System: *Asthma, spasmodic cough.*

Digestive System: *Indigestion, nervous dyspepsia.*

Genitourinary and Endocrine Systems: *Amenorrhea, menstrual cramp, supports female estrogens, promotes feminine characteristics, reduces sexual overactivity.*

Nervous System: *Headaches, insomnia, nervous tension, neuralgia, stress-related conditions.*

EXTRACTION

Essential oil by steam distillation from the dried cones or catkins, known as "strobiles". (An absolute is also produced by solvent extraction for perfumery use.)

ACTIONS

Anodyne, an aphrodisiac, antimicrobial, antiseptic, antispasmodic, astringent, bactericidal, carminative, diuretic, emollient, estrogenic properties, hypnotic, nervine, sedative, soporific.

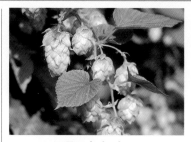

Humulus lupulus

COMPATIBILITIES

It blends well with pine, hyacinth, nutmeg, copaiba, balsam, citrus, and spice oils.

SAFETY DATA
Generally nontoxic (narcotic in excessive amounts) and nonirritant; may cause sensitization in some individuals. Should be avoided by those suffering from depression

HELICHRYSUM ANGUSTIFOLIUM

Helichrysum

FAMILY: ASTERACEAE (COMPOSITAE)

Herbal/Folk Tradition

In Europe it is used for respiratory ailments such as asthma, whooping cough, and chronic bronchitis; also for headaches, migraine, liver ailments, and skin complaints including allergies and psoriasis.

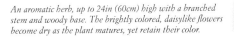

FRESH LEAVES

An aromatic herb, up to 24in (60cm) high with a branched stem and woody base. The brightly colored, daisylike flowers become dry as the plant matures, yet retain their color.

DATAFILE

AROMATHERAPY/ HOME USE

Skin Care: *Abscess, acne, allergic conditions, blemishes, boils, burns, cuts, dermatitis, eczema, inflammation, wounds.*

Circulation, Muscles, and Joints: *Muscular aches and pains, sprains, strains, rheumatism.*

Respiratory System: *Asthma, bronchitis, chronic coughs.*

Digestive System: *Liver congestion, spleen congestion.*

Immune System: *Bacterial infections, colds, flu, fever.*

Nervous System: *Depression, debility, lethargy, neuralgia.*

EXTRACTION

Essential oil by steam distillation from fresh flowers, absolute by solvent extraction.

ACTIONS

Antiallergenic, anti-inflammatory, antimicrobial, antitussive, antiseptic, astringent, cholagogue, cicatrizant, diuretic, hepatic, expectorant, fungicidal, nervine.

COMPATIBILITIES

Citrus oils, chamomile, clove, boronia, labdanum, lavender, mimosa, oakmoss, geranium, clary sage, rose, Peru balsam.

SAFETY DATA

Nontoxic, nonirritant, nonsensitizing

HYACINTHUS ORIENTALIS

Hyacinth

FAMILY: LILIACEAE

Herbal/Folk Tradition

The wild bulbs are poisonous; however, the white juice used to be employed as a substitute for starch or glue. The dried and powdered roots, are balsamic, and believed to have some styptic properties.

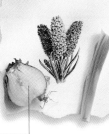

SLICED HYACINTH BULB

A much-loved cultivated plant with fragrant, bell-shaped flowers of many colors, bright lance-shaped leaves, and a round bulb.

DATAFILE

AROMATHERAPY/ HOME USE

Nervous System:

The Greeks described the fragrance of hyacinth as being refreshing and invigorating to a tired mind. It may also be used for stress-related conditions, in self-hypnosis techniques, and in the development of the creative right-hand side of the brain.

EXTRACTION

Concrete and absolute by solvent extraction from the flowers. (An essential oil is also obtained by steam distillation from the absolute.)

ACTIONS

Antiseptic, balsamic, hypnotic, sedative, styptic.

COMPATIBILITIES

It blends well with narcissus, violet, ylang ylang, styrax, galbanum, jasmine, neroli, and with oriental-type bases.

SAFETY DATA

No safety data available at present. Most commercial hyacinth is nowadays adulterated or synthetic

Hyssop

FAMILY: LAMIACEAE (LABIATAE)

Herbal/Folk Tradition

H. officinalis has an ancient medical reputation and was used for purifying sacred places and employed as a strewing herb.

It is used mainly for respiratory and digestive complaints, and externally for rheumatism, bruises, sores, earache, and toothache.

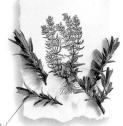

FRESH HYSSOP

An attractive perennial, almost evergreen subshrub up to 24in (60cm) high with a woody stem, small, lance-shaped leaves, and purplish-blue flowers.

DATAFILE

AROMATHERAPY/ HOME USE

Skin Care: *Bruises, cuts, dermatitis, eczema, inflammation, wounds.*

Circulation, Muscles, and Joints: *Low or high blood pressure, rheumatism.*

Respiratory System: *Asthma, bronchitis, catarrh, cough, sore throat, tonsillitis.*

Digestive System: *Colic, indigestion.*

Genitourinary System: *Amenorrhea, leucorrhea.*

Immune System: *Colds, flu.*

Nervous System: *Anxiety, fatigue.*

EXTRACTION

Essential oil by steam distillation from leaves and flowering tops.

ACTIONS

Astringent, antiseptic, antispasmodic, antiviral, bactericidal, carminative, cephalic, cicatrizant, digestive, diuretic, emmenagogue, expectorant, febrifuge, hypertensive, nervine, sedative, sudorific, tonic (heart), vermifuge, vulnerary.

COMPATIBILITIES

Bay leaf, citrus, clary sage, geranium, myrtle, and rosemary.

SAFETY DATA

Nonirritant, nonsensitizing; the oil is moderately toxic due to the pinocamphone content. To be used only in moderation and avoided in pregnancy and by epileptics. Contraindicated in cases of high blood pressure

Star anise

FAMILY: ILLICIACEAE

Herbal/Folk Tradition

Used in Chinese medicine for over 1,300 years for its stimulating effect on the digestive system and for respiratory disorders such as bronchitis and dry coughs.

STAR ANISE SEEDS

DRIED SEED-BEARING FOLLICLES

Evergreen tree up to 39ft (12m) high with a tall, slender white trunk. It bears fruit that consist of five to thirteen seed-bearing follicles attached to a central axis in the shape of a star.

DATAFILE

AROMATHERAPY/ HOME USE

Circulation, Muscles, and Joints: *Muscular aches and pains, rheumatism.*

Respiratory System: *Bronchitis, coughs.*

Digestive System: *Colic, cramp, flatulence, indigestion.*

Immune System: *Colds.*

EXTRACTION

Essential oil by steam distillation from the fruits, fresh or partially dried. An oil is also produced from leaves in small quantities.

ACTIONS

Antiseptic, carminative, expectorant, insect repellent, stimulant.

COMPATIBILITIES

It blends well with rose, lavender, orange, pine, and other spice oils, and has excellent masking properties.

SAFETY DATA

Despite the anethole content, it does not appear to be a dermal irritant, unlike aniseed. In large doses it is narcotic and slows down the circulation; it can lead to cerebral disorders. Use in moderation only. Avoid during pregnancy

INULA HELENIUM

Elecampane

FAMILY: ASTERACEAE (COMPOSITAE)

Herbal/Folk Tradition

An herb that used to be candied and sold as a sweetmeat. It is used for respiratory conditions such as bronchitis, asthma, and whooping cough, disorders of the digestion, intestines, and gall bladder

FRESH
ELECAMPANE

A perennial herb up to 5ft (1.5m) high, with a stout stem covered with soft hairs. It has oval pointed leaves with a velvety underside, yellow flowers, and fleshy rhizome roots.

DATAFILE

AROMATHERAPY/HOME USE
None. NB: Elecampane is a rich source of inulin. Sweet inulin oil is said to have sedative, anti-inflammatory, hyperthermic, cardioregulative, diuretic, and depurative actions. When it is used as an inhalation or by aerosol treatment this variety of Inula avoids the sensitization problems of elecampane, .

EXTRACTION
Essential oil by steam distillation from dried roots and rhizomes.

ACTIONS
Alterative, anthelmintic, anti-inflammatory, antiseptic, antispasmodic, antitussive, astringent, bactericidal, diaphoretic, diuretic, expectorant, fungicidal, hyperglycemic, hypotensive, stomachic, tonic.

COMPATIBILITIES
It blends well with cananga, cinnamon, labdanum, lavender, mimosa, frankincense, orris, tuberose, volet, cedarwood, patchouli, sandalwood, cypress, bergamot, and oriental fragrances.

SAFETY DATA
Nontoxic, nonirritant, a severe dermal sensitizer. In clinical tests it caused "extremely severe allergic reactions" in 23 out of 25 volunteers; therefore, it is recommended that the oil "should not be used on the skin at all"[15]

IRIS PALLIDA

Orris

FAMILY: IRIDACEAE

Herbal/Folk Tradition

In ancient Greece and Rome orris root was used extensively in perfumery, and its medicinal qualities were held in high esteem. It was once used for upper respiratory tract catarrh, coughs, and for diarrhea in infants.

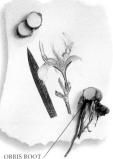

ORRIS ROOT

A decorative perennial plant up to 5ft (1.5m) high, with sword-shaped leaves, a creeping fleshy rootstock, and delicate, scented, pale blue flowers.

DATAFILE

AROMATHERAPY/HOME USE
None. However, the powdered orris, which is a common article, may be used as a dry shampoo, a body powder, a fixative for pot-pourris, and to scent linen.

EXTRACTION
A concrete is produced by steam distillation from the rhizomes that have been peeled, washed, dried, and pulverized. Rhizomes must be stored for at least three years otherwise they have virtually no scent. An absolute is produced by alkali washing in ethyl ether solution to remove the myristic acid from the concrete oil. A resin or resinoid is produced by alcohol extraction from the peeled rhizomes.

ACTIONS
Dried root – antidiarrheal, demulcent, expectorant. Fresh root – diuretic, cathartic, emetic.

COMPATIBILITIES
It blends well with cedarwood, sandalwood, vetiver, cypress, mimosa, labdanum, bergamot, clary sage, rose, violet and other florals.

SAFETY DATA
The fresh root causes nausea and vomiting in large doses. The oil and absolute are much adulterated or synthetic – "true" orris absolute is three times the price of jasmine

JASMINUM OFFICINALE

Jasmine

FAMILY: OLEACEAE

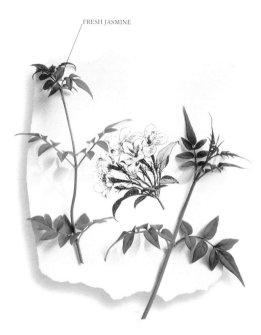

FRESH JASMINE

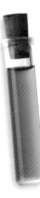

Herbal/Folk Tradition

In China the flowers of *J. officinale var. grandiflorum* are used to treat hepatitis, liver cirrhosis, and dysentery; the flowers of *J. sambac* are used for conjunctivitis, dysentery, skin ulcers, and tumors. The root is used to treat headaches, insomnia, pain due to dislocated joints and rheumatism.

In the West, the common jasmine was said in Culpeper's *Complete Herbal* to "warm the womb … and facilitate the birth; it is useful for cough, difficulty of breathing, etc. It disperses crude humours, and is good for cold and catarrhous constitutions, but not for the hot."[16] It was also used for hard, contracted limbs and problems with the nervous and reproductive systems.

An evergreen shrub or vine up to 33ft (10m) high with delicate, bright green leaves and star-shaped very fragrant white flowers.

DATAFILE

AROMATHERAPY/ HOME USE

Skin Care: *Dry, greasy, irritated, sensitive skin.*
Circulation, Muscles, and Joints: *Muscular spasm, sprains.*
Respiratory System: *Catarrh, coughs, hoarseness, laryngitis.*
Genitourinary System: *Dysmenorrhea, frigidity, labor pains, uterine disorders.*
Nervous System: *Depression, nervous exhaustion and stress-related conditions.* "It ... produces *a feeling of optimism, confidence and euphoria. It is most useful in cases where there is apathy, indifference, or listlessness.*"[17]

EXTRACTION

A concrete is produced by solvent extraction; the absolute is obtained from the concrete by separation with alcohol. An essential oil is produced by steam distillation of the absolute.

ACTIONS

Analgesic (mild), antidepressant, anti-inflammatory, antiseptic, antispasmodic, aphrodisiac, carminative, cicatrizant, expectorant, galactagogue, parturient, sedative, tonic (uterine).

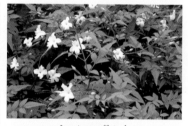

Jasminum officinale

COMPATIBILITIES

It blends well with rose, sandalwood, clary sage, and all the citrus oils. It has the ability to round off any rough notes and blend with virtually everything.

SAFETY DATA
Nontoxic, nonirritant, generally nonsensitizing (an allergic reaction has been known to occur in some individuals)

JUNIPERUS ASHEI

Texas cedarwood

FAMILY: CUPRESSACEAE

Herbal/Folk Tradition

In New Mexico the Native Americans use cedarwood oil for skin rashes. It is also used for arthritis and rheumatism.

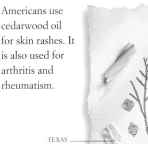

TEXAS CEDARWOOD CHIPPINGS

A small, alpine evergreen tree up to 23ft (7m) high with stiff green needles and an irregular-shaped trunk and branches, which tend to be crooked or twisted. The wood also tends to crack easily, so it is not used for lumber.

DATAFILE

AROMATHERAPY/ HOME USE

Skin Care: *Acne, dandruff, eczema, greasy hair, insect repellent, oily skin, psoriasis.*

Circulation, Muscles, and Joints: *Arthritis, rheumatism.*

Respiratory System: *Bronchitis, catarrh, congestion, coughs, sinusitis.*

Genitourinary System: *Cystitis, leucorrhea.*

Nervous System: *Nervous tension and stress-related disorders.*

EXTRACTION

Essential oil by steam distillation from the heartwood and wood shavings, etc.

ACTIONS

Antiseptic, antispasmodic, astringent, diuretic, expectorant, sedative (nervous), stimulant (circulatory).

COMPATIBILITIES

Rectified oil blends well with patchouli, spruce, vetiver, pine, and leather-type scents.

SAFETY DATA

Externally the oil is relatively nontoxic; it can cause acute local irritation and possible sensitization in some. Use in dilution only with care, in moderation. Avoid during pregnancy. Generally safer to use Atlas cedarwood

---

JUNIPERUS COMMUNIS

Juniper

FAMILY: CUPRESSACEAE

Herbal/Folk Tradition

Used medicinally for urinary infections, for respiratory problems, as well as gastrointestinal infections and worms. It helps expel the buildup of uric acid in the joints and is employed in gout, rheumatism, and arthritis.

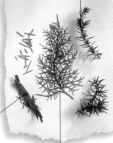

FLOWERS

BARK AND NEEDLES

JUNIPER BERRIES

An evergreen shrub or tree up to 20ft (6m) high, with bluish-green stiff needles. It has small flowers and berries that are green in the first year, black in the second and third.

DATAFILE

AROMATHERAPY/ HOME USE

Skin Care: *Acne, dermatitis, eczema, hair loss, hemorrhoids, oily complexions, wounds.*

Circulation, Muscles, and Joints: *Arteriosclerosis, cellulitis, gout, obesity, rheumatism.*

Immune System: *Colds, flu.*

Genitourinary System: *Amenorrhea, cystitis, dysmenorrhea, leucorrhea.*

Nervous System: *Anxiety, tension*

EXTRACTION

Essential oil by steam distillation of the berries, needles and wood.

ACTIONS

Antirheumatic, antiseptic, antispasmodic, antitoxic, aphrodisiac, astringent, carminative, cicatrizant, depurative, diuretic, emmenagogue, nervine, parasiticide, rubefacient, sedative, stomachic, sudorific, vulnerary.

COMPATIBILITIES

Vetiver, sandalwood, cedarwood, mastic, oakmoss, galbanum, elemi, cypress, clary sage, pine, lavender, lavandin, labdanum, fir needle, rosemary, benzoin, balsam tolu, geranium, and citrus oils.

SAFETY DATA

Nonsensitizing, may be slightly irritating, nontoxic. Stimulates the uterine muscle and must not be used during pregnancy. Should not be used by those with kidney disease due to its nephrotoxic effect. Use only juniper berry oil, in moderation

JUNIPERUS OXYCEDRUS

Cade

FAMILY: CUPRESSACEAE

Herbal/Folk Tradition

Used in the treatment of cutaneous diseases, such as chronic eczema, parasites, scalp disease, hair loss, etc., especially in France and other European countries. It is also used as an antiseptic wound dressing and for toothache.

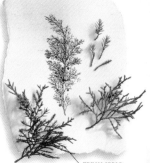

FRESH SPRIG

CADE NEEDLES

A large evergreen shrub up to 13ft (4m) high, with long dark needles and brownish-black berries about the size of hazelnuts.

DATAFILE	
AROMATHERAPY/ HOME USE Skin Care: *Cuts, blemishes, dandruff, dermatitis, eczema, etc.* **EXTRACTION** The crude oil or tar is obtained by destructive distillation from the branches and heartwood (usually in the form of shavings or chips). A rectified oil is produced from the crude by steam or vacuum distillation. An oil is sometimes produced from the berries by steam distillation.	**ACTIONS** Analgesic, antimicrobial, antipruritic, antiseptic, disinfectant, parasiticide, vermifuge. **COMPATIBILITIES** It blends well with thyme, origanum, clove, cassia, tea tree, pine, and medicinal bases.

SAFETY DATA
Nontoxic, nonirritant, possible sensitization problems. Use with care, especially when treating inflammatory or allergic skin conditions. Turpentine (terebinth) oil makes a useful alternative, with less possibility of an allergic reaction

---

JUNIPERUS SABINA

Savine

FAMILY: CUPRESSACEAE

Herbal/Folk Tradition

It was used at one time as an ointment or dressing for blisters, in order to promote discharge, and for syphilitic warts and other skin problems. It should never be used in pregnancy.

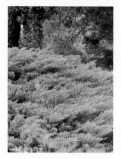

FRESH SPRIG

A compact evergreen shrub about 3ft (1m) high (much taller around the Mediterranean), which tends to spread horizontally. It has a pale green bark, small, dark green leaves, and purplish-black berries containing three seeds.

DATAFILE	
AROMATHERAPY/ HOME USE None. Should not be used in therapy, whether internally or externally. **EXTRACTION** Essential oil by steam distillation from the twigs and leaves. **ACTIONS** Powerful anthelmintic, diuretic, emmenagogue, rubefacient, stimulant, vermifuge.	*Juniperus sabina* *Native to North America, middle and southern Europe. The oil is produced mainly in Austria.*

SAFETY DATA
Oral toxin. Dermal irritant. Abortifacient. "The oil is banned from sale to the public in many countries due to its toxic effects (nerve poison and blood circulation stimulant)."[18]

JUNIPERUS VIRGINIANA

Virginian cedarwood

FAMILY: CUPRESSACEAE

Herbal/Folk Tradition

The Native Americans used it for respiratory infections. Decoctions of leaves, bark, twigs, and fruit were used to treat kidney infections, menstrual delay, gonorrhea, rheumatism, arthritis, skin rashes, venereal warts.

FRESH VIRGINIAN CEDARWOOD

A coniferous, slow-growing, evergreen tree up to 108ft (33m) high with a narrow, dense, and pyramidal crown, a reddish heartwood, and brown cones. The trunk diameter can reach over 5ft (1.5m).

DATAFILE

AROMATHERAPY/ HOME USE
Skin Care: *Acne, dandruff, eczema, greasy hair, insect repellent, oily skin, psoriasis.*
Circulation, Muscles, and Joints: *Arthritis, rheumatism.*
Respiratory System: *Bronchitis, catarrh, congestion, coughs, sinusitis.*
Genitourinary System: *Cystitis, leucorrhea.*
Nervous System: *Nervous tension and stress-related disorders.*

EXTRACTION
Essential oil by steam distillation from the timber waste.

ACTIONS
Abortifacient, antiseborrheic, antiseptic (pulmonary, genito-urinary), antispasmodic, astringent, balsamic, diuretic, emmenagogue, expectorant, insecticide, sedative (nervous), stimulant (circulatory).

COMPATIBILITIES
It blends well with benzoin, sandalwood, rose, juniper, cypress, vetiver, and patchouli.

SAFETY DATA
See Texas cedarwood, page 93

LAURUS NOBILIS

Bay laurel

FAMILY: LAURACEAE

Herbal/Folk Tradition

A popular culinary herb throughout Europe. Both leaf and berry were formerly used for a variety of afflictions including hysteria, colic, indigestion, loss of appetite, to promote menstruation, and for fever.

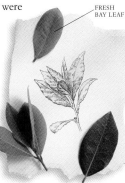

FRESH BAY LEAF

An evergreen tree up to 65ft (20m) high with dark green, glossy leaves and black berries; often cultivated as an ornamental shrub.

DATAFILE

AROMATHERAPY/ HOME USE
Digestive System: *Dyspepsia, flatulence, loss of appetite.*
Genitourinary System: *Scanty periods.*
Immune System: *Colds, flu, tonsillitis, and viral infections.*

EXTRACTION
Essential oil by steam distillation from the dried leaf and branchlets. An oil from the berries is produced in small quantities.

ACTIONS
Antirheumatic, antiseptic, bactericidal, diaphoretic, digestive, diuretic, emmenagogue, fungicidal, hypotensive, sedative, stomachic.

COMPATIBILITIES
It blends well with pine, cypress, juniper, clary sage, rosemary, olibanum, labdanum, lavender, citrus and spice oils.

SAFETY DATA
Relatively nontoxic and nonirritant; can cause dermatitis in some individuals. Use in moderation due to possible narcotic properties attributed to methyl eugenol. Should not be used during pregnancy

LAVANDULA ANGUSTIFOLIA

LAVANDULA ANGUSTIFOLIA

True lavender

FAMILY: LAMIACEAE (LABIATAE)

Herbal/Folk Tradition

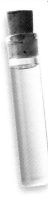

Lavender has a well-established tradition as a folk remedy, and its scent is still familiar to almost everyone. It was used to "comfort the stomach" but above all as a cosmetic water, an insect repellent, to scent linen, and as a reviving yet soothing oil. Generally regarded as the most versatile essence therapeutically.

FRESH LAVENDER

An evergreen woody shrub, up to 3ft (1m) tall, with pale green, narrow, linear leaves and flowers on blunt spikes of a beautiful violet-blue color. The whole plant is highly aromatic.

DATAFILE

AROMATHERAPY/ HOME USE

Skin Care: *Abscesses, acne, allergies, athlete's foot, blemishes, all skin types, boils, bruises, burns, dandruff, dermatitis, earache, eczema, inflammations, insect bites and stings, insect repellent, lice, psoriasis, ringworm, scabies, sores, sunburn, wounds.*
Circulation, Muscles, and Joints: *Lumbago, muscular aches and pains, rheumatism, sprains.*
Respiratory System: *Asthma, bronchitis, catarrh, halitosis, laryngitis, throat infections, whooping cough.*

Digestive System: *Abdominal cramps, colic, dyspepsia, flatulence, nausea.*
Genitourinary System: *Cystitis, dysmenorrhea, leucorrhea.*
Immune System: *Flu.*
Nervous System: *Depression, headache, hypertension, insomnia, migraine, nervous tension and stress-related conditions, PMS, sciatica, shock, vertigo.*

EXTRACTION

Essential oil by steam distillation from the fresh flowering tops. An absolute and concrete are also produced by solvent extraction in smaller quantities.

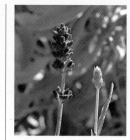

Lavandula angustifolia

ACTIONS

Analgesic, anticonvulsive, antidepressant, antimicrobial, antirheumatic, antiseptic, antispasmodic, antitoxic, carminative, cholagogue, choleretic, cicatrizant, cordial, cytophylactic, deodorant, diuretic, emmenagogue, hypotensive, insecticide, nervine, parasiticide, rubefacient, sedative, stimulant, sudorific, tonic, vermifuge, vulnerary.

COMPATIBILITIES

It blends well with most oils, especially citrus and florals; also cedarwood, clove, clary sage, pine, geranium, labdanum, oakmoss, vetiver, and patchouli.

SAFETY DATA

Nontoxic, nonirritant, nonsensitizing

LAVANDULA X INTERMEDIA

Lavandin

FAMILY: LAMIACEAE (LABIATAE)

Herbal/Folk Tradition

Sixty years ago lavandin was still unknown, so it does not have a long history of therapeutic use. Its properties seem to combine those of the true lavender and aspic.

FRESH
LAVANDIN LEAF

A hybrid plant developed by crossing true lavender (L. angustifolia) *with spike lavender or aspic* (L. latifolia). *In general, it is a larger plant than true lavender, with woody stems. Its flowers may be blue, or grayish like aspic.*

**AROMATHERAPY/
HOME USE**
Similar uses to true lavender, but it is more penetrating and rubefacient with a sharper scent – good for respiratory, circulatory, or muscular conditions.

EXTRACTION
Essential oil by steam distillation from the fresh flowering tops; it has a higher yield of oil than either true lavender or apic. (A concrete and absolute are produced by solvent extraction.)

ACTIONS
See True lavender, page 96.

COMPATIBILITIES
It blends well with clove, bay leaf, cinnamon, citronella, cypress, pine, clary sage, geranium, thyme, patchouli, rosemary, and citrus oils, especially bergamot and lime.

SAFETY DATA
Nontoxic, nonirritant, nonsensitizing

LAVANDULA LATIFOLIA

Spike lavender

FAMILY: LAMIACEAE (LABIATAE)

Herbal/Folk Tradition

Culpeper recommends spike lavender for "pains of the head and brain which proceed from cold, apoplexy, falling sickness, the dropsy, or sluggish malady, cramps, convulsions, palsies, and often faintings."[19]

FRESH LEAVES

An aromatic evergreen subshrub up to 3ft (1m) high with lance-shaped leaves, broader and rougher than those of true lavender. The flower is more compressed and of a dull gray-blue color.

**AROMATHERAPY/
HOME USE**
See True lavender, page 96.

EXTRACTION
Essential oil by water or steam distillation from the flowering tops

ACTIONS
See True lavender, page 96.

COMPATIBILITIES
It blends well with rosemary, sage, lavandin, eucalyptus, rosewood, lavender, petitgrain, pine, cedarwood, oakmoss, patchouli, and spice oils, particularly clove.

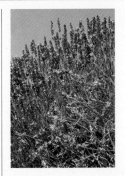

Lavandula latifolia

SAFETY DATA
Nontoxic, nonirritant (except in concentration), nonsensitizing

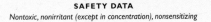

Lovage

FAMILY: APIACEAE (UMBELLIFERAE)

Herbal/Folk Tradition

A herb of ancient medical repute, used mainly for digestive complaints, edema, skin problems, menstrual irregularities, and fever. It was also believed to be good for the sight. The leaf stalks used to be blanched and used as a vegetable or in salads. The root is current in the British Herbal Pharmacopoeia as a specific for flatulent dyspepsia and anorexia.

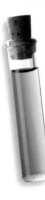

The oil obtained from the fresh roots is amber or olive-brown, with a rich spicy, warm, rootlike odor.

FRESH LOVAGE

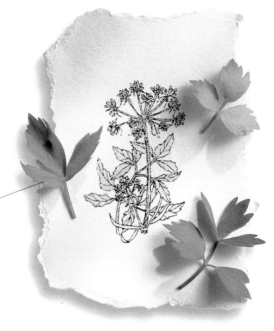

A large perennial herb up to 6ft (2m) high with a stout hollow stem and dense ornamental foliage. It has a thick fleshy root and greenish-yellow flowers. The whole plant has a strong aromatic scent.

DATAFILE

AROMATHERAPY/ HOME USE

Circulation, Muscles, and Joints: *Accumulation of toxins, congestion, gout, edema, poor circulation, rheumatism, water retention.*

Digestive System: *Anemia, flatulence, indigestion, spasm.*

Genitourinary System: *Amenorrhea, dysmenorrhea, cystitis.*

EXTRACTION

Essential oil by steam distillation from the fresh roots and the fresh leaves and stalks of the herb.

ACTIONS

Antimicrobial, antiseptic, antispasmodic, diaphoretic, digestive, diuretic, carminative, depurative, emmenagogue, expectorant, febrifuge, stimulant (digestive), stomachic.

COMPATIBILITIES

It blends well with rose, galbanum, costus, opopanax, oakmoss, bay, lavandin, and spice oils.

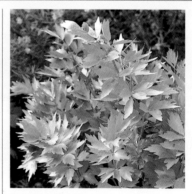

Levisticum officinale

SAFETY DATA
Nontoxic, nonirritant, possible sensitization/phototoxic effects. Use with care. Avoid during pregnancy

LIQUIDAMBAR ORIENTALIS

Levant styrax

FAMILY: HAMAMELIDACEAE

Herbal/Folk Tradition

In China it is used for coughs, colds, epilepsy, and skin problems, including cuts, wounds, and scabies. It is recommended in the West for catarrh, diphtheria, gonorrhea, leucorrhea, and ringworm.

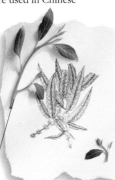

FRESH LEAVES

A deciduous tree, up to 49ft (15m) high, with a purplish-gray bark, leaves arranged into five three-lobed sections, and white flowers. Styrax is produced by pounding the bark, which induces the sapwood to produce a liquid.

DATAFILE	
AROMATHERAPY/ HOME USE	**ACTIONS**
Skin Care: *Cuts, ringworm, scabies, wounds.*	Anti-inflammatory, antimicrobial, antiseptic, antitussive, bactericidal, balsamic, expectorant, nervine, stimulant.
Respiratory System: *Bronchitis, catarrh, coughs.*	
Nervous System: *Anxiety, stress-related conditions.*	
	COMPATIBILITIES
EXTRACTION	It blends well with ylang ylang, jasmine, mimosa, rose, lavender, carnation, violet, cassie, and spice oils.
Essential oil by steam distillation from the crude. A resinoid and absolute are also produced by solvent extraction.	

SAFETY DATA
Nontoxic, nonirritant, possible sensitization in some individuals. Frequently adulterated

---

LITSEA CUBEBA

Litsea cubeba

FAMILY: LAURACEAE

Herbal/Folk Tradition

The root and stem are used in Chinese medicine to treat dysmenorrhea, indigestion, lower back pain, chills, headaches, travel sickness, and muscle aches. It may be valuable in treating arrythmia.

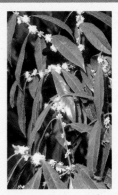

FRESH LITSEA CUBEBA

Litsea cubeba

A small tropical tree with fragrant, lemongrass-scented leaves and flowers. The small fruits are shaped like peppers, from which the name "cubeba" derives.

DATAFILE
AROMATHERAPY/ HOME USE
Skin Care: *Acne, dermatitis, insect repellent, profuse perspiration, .*
Digestive System: *Flatulence, indigestion.*
Immune System: *Sanitation.*
Nervous System: *Arrhythmia, high blood pressure, nervous tension, and stress-related conditions.*
EXTRACTION
Essential oil by steam distillation from the fruits.
ACTIONS
Antiseptic, deodorant, digestive, disinfectant, insecticidal, sedative, stomachic.

SAFETY DATA
Nontoxic, nonirritant, possible sensitization in some individuals

MATRICARIA RECUTICA

German chamomile

FAMILY: ASTERACEAE (COMPOSITAE)

Herbal/Folk Tradition

This herb has a long-standing medicinal tradition, especially in Europe. An excellent skin care remedy, it has greater anti-inflammatory properties than Roman chamomile.

GERMAN
CHAMOMILE
SEEDS

**AROMATHERAPY/
HOME USE**
See Roman chamomile, page 64.

EXTRACTION
Essential oil by steam distillation from the flowerheads (up to 1.9 per cent yield). An absolute is also produced in small quantities, which is a deeper blue color and has greater tenacity and fixative properties.

ACTIONS
Analgesic, antiallergenic, anti-inflammatory, antiphlogistic, antispasmodic, bactericidal, carminative, cicatrizant, cholagogue, digestive, emmenagogue, febrifuge, fungicidal, hepatic, nerve sedative, stimulant of leucocyte production, stomachic, sudorific, vermifuge, vulnerary.

COMPATIBILITIES
It blends well with geranium, lavender, patchouli, rose, benzoin, neroli, bergamot, marjoram, lemon, ylang ylang, jasmine, clary sage, and labdanum.

SAFETY DATA
Nontoxic, nonirritant, causes dermatitis in some individuals

An annual, strongly aromatic herb, up to 24in (60cm) tall, with a hairless, erect, branching stem. It has feathery leaves and simple daisylike white flowers on single stems.

MELALEUCA CAJEPUTI

Cajeput

FAMILY: MYRTACEAE

FRESH
CAJEPUT

Herbal/Folk Tradition

In the East, it is used locally for colds, headaches, throat infections, toothache, sore muscles, fever rheumatism and various skin diseases. In the West the oil is known for producing a sensation of warmth.

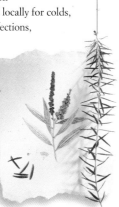

**AROMATHERAPY/
HOME USE**
Skin Care: *Blemishes, insect bites, oily skin.*
Circulation, Muscles, and Joints: *Arthritis, muscular aches and pains, rheumatism.*
Respiratory System: *Asthma, bronchitis, catarrh, coughs, sinusitis, sore throat.*
Genitourinary System: *Cystitis, urethritis, urinary infection.*
Immune System:
Colds, flu, viral infections.

EXTRACTION
Essential oil by steam distillation from the fresh leaves and twigs.

ACTIONS
Mildly analgesic, antimicrobial, antineuralgic, antispasmodic, antiseptic (pulmonary, urinary, intestinal), anthelmintic, diaphoretic, carminative, expectorant, febrifuge, insecticide, sudorific, tonic.

SAFETY DATA
Nontoxic, nonsensitizing, may irritate the skin in high concentration

An evergreen tree up to 98ft (30m) high, with thick pointed leaves and white flowers. The flexible trunk has a whitish spongy bark that flakes off easily.

MELALEUCA ALTERNIFOLIA

Tea tree

FAMILY: MYRTACEAE

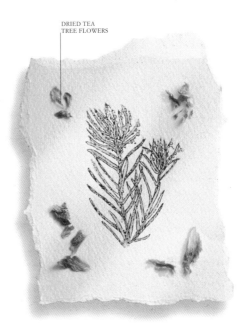

DRIED TEA
TREE FLOWERS

Herbal/Folk Tradition

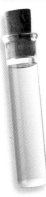

The name derives from its local usage as a type of herbal tea, prepared from the leaves. Our present knowledge of tea tree is based on a very long history of use by the aboriginal people of Australia. It has been extensively researched by scientific methods with the following results: "1. This oil is unusual in that it is active against all three varieties of infectious organisms: bacteria, fungi, and viruses. 2. It is a very powerful immuno-stimulant, so when the body is threatened by any of these organisms ti-tree increases its ability to respond."[20]

A small tree or shrub (smallest of the tea tree family), with needle-like leaves similar to cypress, with heads of sessile yellow or purplish flowers.

DATAFILE

AROMATHERAPY/ HOME USE

Skin Care: *Abscess, acne, athlete's foot, blemishes, blisters, burns, cold sores, dandruff, herpes, insect bites, oily skin, plantar warts (verrucae), rashes (diaper rash), warts, wounds (infected).*
Respiratory System: *Asthma, bronchitis, catarrh, coughs, sinusitis, tuberculosis, whooping cough.*
Genitourinary System: *Thrush, vaginitis, cystitis, pruritis.*
Immune System: *Colds, fever, flu, infectious illnesses such as chickenpox.*

EXTRACTION

Essential oil by distillation (steam) from leaves and twigs.

ACTIONS

Anti-infectious, anti-inflammatory, antiseptic, antiviral, bactericidal, balsamic, cicatrizant, diaphoretic, expectorant, fungicidal, immunostimulant, parasiticide, vulnerary.

COMPATIBILITIES

Lavandin, lavender, clary sage, rosemary, oakmoss, pine, cananga, geranium, marjoram, and spice oils,

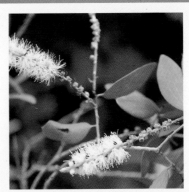

Melaleuca alternifolia

SAFETY DATA
Nontoxic, nonirritant, possible sensitization in some individuals

---

MELALEUCA VIRIDIFLORA

Niaouli

FAMILY: MYRTACEAE

Herbal/Folk Tradition

Native to Australia, New Caledonia, and the French Pacific Islands, it is used locally for a wide variety of ailments, such as aches and pains, respiratory conditions, cuts, and infections; it is also used to purify water.

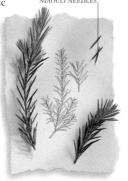

NIAOULI NEEDLES

An evergreen tree with a flexible trunk and spongy bark, pointed linear leaves, and spikes of sessile yellowish flowers. The leaves have a strong aromatic scent when crushed.

DATAFILE

AROMATHERAPY/ HOME USE

Skin Care: *Acne, blemishes, boils, burns, cuts, insect bites, oily skin, ulcers, wounds.*
Circulation, Muscles, and Joints: *Muscular aches and pains, poor circulation, rheumatism.*
Respiratory System: *Asthma, bronchitis, catarrhal conditions, coughs, sinusitis, sore throat, whooping cough.*
Genitourinary System: *Cystitis, urinary infection.*
Immune System: *Colds, fever, flu.*

EXTRACTION

Essential oil by steam distillation from the leaves and young twigs. (Usually rectified to remove irritant aldehydes.)

ACTIONS

Analgesic, anthelmintic, anticatarrhal, antirheumatic, antiseptic, antispasmodic, bactericidal, balsamic, cicatrizant, diaphoretic, expectorant, regulator, stimulant, vermifuge.

SAFETY DATA

Nontoxic, nonirritant, nonsensitizing. Often subject to adulteration

---

MELILOTUS OFFICINALIS

Melilotus

FAMILY: FABACEAE (LEGUMINOSAE)

Herbal/Folk Tradition

The leaves and shoots are used in continental Europe for conditions that include sleeplessness, thrombosis, tension, varicose veins, intestinal disorders, headache, and earache.

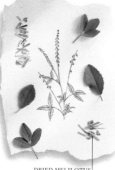

DRIED MELILOTUS

A bushy perennial herb up to 3ft (1m) high, with smooth erect stems, trifoliate oval leaves, and small sweet-scented white or yellow flowers – their scent is stronger on drying.

DATAFILE

AROMATHERAPY/ HOME USE
None.

EXTRACTION
A concrete (usually called a resinoid or oleoresin) by solvent extraction from the dry flowers

ACTIONS
Anti-inflammatory, antirheumatic, antispasmodic, astringent, emollient, expectorant, digestive, insecticidal (against moth), sedative.

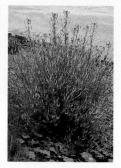

Melilotus officinalis
Native to Europe and Asia
Minor. The oleoresin is used in
high-quality perfumery work.

SAFETY DATA
In 1953 in some countries, including the United States, coumarin was banned from use in flavorings due to toxicity levels. Some coumarins are also known to be phototoxic.

MELISSA OFFICINALIS

Lemon balm

FAMILY: LAMIACEAE (LABIATAE)

Herbal/Folk Tradition

One of the earliest known medicinal herbs, associated with nervous disorders, the heart, and the emotions. It is generally used for respiratory and digestive complaints of nervous origin such as asthma, indigestion, and flatulence.

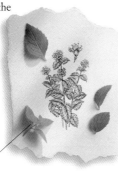

FRESH LEAVES

A sweet-scented herb about 24in (60cm) high, soft and bushy, with bright green serrated leaves, square stems, and tiny white or pink flowers.

DATAFILE	
AROMATHERAPY/ HOME USE	**EXTRACTION**
Skin Care: *Allergies, insect bites and repellent. Low concentrations can be used to treat eczema and other skin problems.*	Essential oil by steam distillation from leaves and flowering tops.
Respiratory System: *Asthma, bronchitis, chronic coughs.*	**ACTIONS**
Digestive System: *Colic, indigestion, nausea.*	Antidepressant, antihistaminic, antispasmodic, bactericidal, carminative, cordial, diaphoretic, emmenagogue, febrifuge, hypertensive, nervine, sedative, stomachic, sudorific, tonic, uterine, vermifuge.
Genitourinary System: *Menstrual problems.*	
Nervous System: *Anxiety, depression, hypertension, insomnia, migraine, nervous tension, shock, and vertigo.*	**COMPATIBILITIES** It blends well with lavender, geranium, floral and citrus oils.

SAFETY DATA
Nontoxic. Possible sensitization and dermal irritation: use in low dilutions only. One of the most frequently adulterated oils. Most commercial so-called melissa contains some or all of the following: lemon, lemongrass, or citronella

---

MENTHA ARVENSIS

Cornmint

FAMILY: LAMIACEAE (LABIATAE)

Herbal/Folk Tradition

Used therapeutically in many of the same ways as peppermint. In the East it is used to treat rheumatic pain, neuralgia, toothache, laryngitis, indigestion, colds, and bronchitis.

FRESH CORNMINT LEAVES

A somewhat fragile herb with leafy stems up to 24in (60cm) high, lance-shaped leaves and lilac-colored flowers borne in clustered whorls in the axils of the upper leaves.

DATAFILE	
AROMATHERAPY/ HOME USE	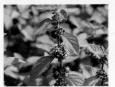
Not compatible with homeopathic treatment. Use Peppermint, see page 104, in preference, since it is not fractionated like the commercial cornmint oil and has a more refined fragrance.	*Mentha arvensis Native to Europe, Japan, and China, and naturalized in North America.*
EXTRACTION Essential oil by steam distillation from the flowering herb. The oil is usually dementholized since it contains so much menthol that it is otherwise solid at room temperature.	**ACTIONS** Anesthetic, antimicrobial, antiseptic, antispasmodic, carminative, cytotoxic, digestive, expectorant, stimulant, stomachic.

SAFETY DATA
Nontoxic, nonirritant (except in concentration); may cause sensitization in some individuals. Menthol is a dermal irritant.

MENTHA PIPERITA

Peppermint

FAMILY: LAMIACEAE (LABIATAE)

FRESH PEPPERMINT LEAVES

Herbal/Folk Tradition

Mints have been cultivated since ancient times in China and Japan. In Egypt evidence of a type of peppermint has been found in tombs dating from 1000 BCE. It has been used extensively in Eastern and Western medicine for a variety of complaints, including indigestion, nausea, sore throat, diarrhea, headaches, toothaches, and cramp. It is current in the British Herbal Pharmacopoeia for intestinal colic, flatulence, common cold, vomiting in pregnancy, and dysmenorrhea.

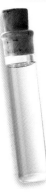

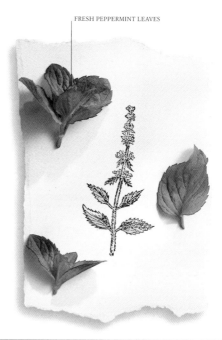

A perennial herb up to 3ft (1m) high with underground runners by which it is easily propagated. The "white" peppermint has green stems and leaves; the "black" peppermint has dark green serrated leaves, purplish stems, and reddish-violet flowers.

DATAFILE

AROMATHERAPY/ HOME USE

Not compatible with homeopathic treatment.

Skin Care: *Acne, dermatitis, ringworm, scabies, toothache.*

Circulation, Muscles, and Joints: *Neuralgia, muscular pain, palpitations.*

Respiratory System: *Asthma, bronchitis, halitosis, sinusitis, spasmodic cough – "When inhaled (in steam) it checks catarrh temporarily, and will provide relief from head colds and bronchitis: its antispasmodic action combines well with this to make it a most useful inhalation in asthma."[21]*

Digestive System: *Colic, cramp, dyspepsia, flatulence, nausea.*

Immune System: *Colds, flu, fevers.*

Nervous System: *Fainting, headache, mental fatigue, migraine, nervous stress, vertigo.*

EXTRACTION

Essential oil by steam distillation from the flowering herb (approx. 3–4 per cent yield).

Mentha piperita

ACTIONS

Analgesic, anti-inflammatory, antimicrobial, antiphlogistic, antipruritic, antiseptic, antispasmodic, antiviral, astringent, carminative, cephalic, cholagogue, cordial, emmenagogue, expectorant, febrifuge, hepatic, nervine, stomachic, sudorific, vasoconstrictor, vermifuge.

COMPATIBILITIES

It blends well with benzoin, rosemary, lavender, marjoram, lemon, eucalyptus, and other mints.

SAFETY DATA

Nontoxic, nonirritant (except in concentration), possible sensitization due to menthol. Use in moderation

MENTHA PULEGIUM

Pennyroyal

FAMILY: LAMIACEAE (LABIATAE)

Herbal/Folk Tradition

A herbal remedy of ancient repute, used for a wide variety of ailments.
It was believed to purify the blood and be able to communicate its purifying qualities to water.

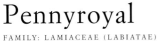

DRIED PENNYROYAL

A perennial herb up to 20in (50cm) tall with smooth roundish stalks, small pale purple flowers, and aromatic, gray-green oval leaves. It has a fibrous creeping root.

DATAFILE

AROMATHERAPY/ HOME USE
None. It should not be used in aromatherapy, either internally or externally.

EXTRACTION
Essential oil by steam distillation from the fresh or slightly dried herb.

ACTIONS
Antiseptic, antispasmodic, diaphoretic, carminative, digestive, emmenagogue, insect repellent, refrigerant, stimulant.

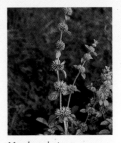

Mentha pulegium

COMPATIBILITIES
It blends well with geranium, rosemary, lavandin, sage, and citronella.

SAFETY DATA
Oral toxin. Abortifacient (due to pulegone content). Ingestion of large doses has resulted in death

MENTHA SPICATA

Spearmint

FAMILY: LAMIACEAE (LABIATAE)

Herbal/Folk Tradition

Valued all over the world as a culinary herb. The ancient Greeks used it to scent their bathwater. The distilled water is used to relieve hiccups, colic, nausea, indigestion, and flatulence.

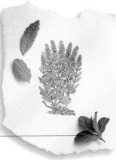

FRESH SPEARMINT

A hardy branched perennial herb with bright green, lance-shaped, sharply serrated leaves, quickly spreading underground runners, and pink or lilac-colored flowers in slender cylindrical spikes.

DATAFILE

AROMATHERAPY/ HOME USE
Not compatible with homeopathic treatment. Less powerful than peppermint oil, it is useful for the treatment of children's maladies.
Skin Care: *Acne, dermatitis, congested skin.*
Respiratory System: *Asthma, bronchitis, catarrhal conditions, sinusitis.*
Digestive System: *Colic, dyspepsia, flatulence, hepatobiliary disorders, nausea.*
Immune System: *Colds, fevers.*
Nervous System: *Fatigue, headache, migraine, nervous strain, neurasthenia, stress.*

EXTRACTION
Essential oil by steam distillation from the flowering tops.

ACTIONS
Anesthetic (local), antiseptic, antispasmodic, astringent, carminative, cephalic, cholagogue, decongestant, digestive, diuretic, expectorant, febrifuge, hepatic, nervine, stimulant, stomachic, tonic.

COMPATIBILITIES
It blends well with lavender, lavandin, jasmine, eucalyptus, basil, and rosemary and is often used in combination with peppermint.

SAFETY DATA
Nontoxic, nonirritant, nonsensitizing

105

MYRISTICA FRAGRANS

Nutmeg

FAMILY: MYRISTICACEAE

Herbal/Folk Tradition

Nutmeg and mace are widely used as domestic spices and have been used for centuries as a remedy for kidney and digestive problems. Grated nutmeg with lard is used for piles. A fixed oil of nutmeg is also used in soap and candle-making.

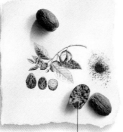

DRIED NUTMEG SEED

Evergreen tree up to 65ft (20m) high with a grayish-brown smooth bark, dense foliage, and small dull-yellow flowers.

DATAFILE	
AROMATHERAPY/ HOME USE Use in moderation, and with care in pregnancy. **Circulation, Muscles, and Joints:** *Arthritis, gout, muscular aches and pains, poor circulation, rheumatism.* **Digestive System:** *Flatulence, indigestion, nausea.* **Immune System:** *Bacterial infection.* **Nervous System:** *Frigidity, impotence, neuralgia, fatigue.* **EXTRACTION** Essential oil by steam (or water) distillation from the dried seed,	or the husk (mace). Oleoresin by solvent extraction from mace. **ACTIONS** Analgesic, antiemetic, antioxidant, antirheumatic, antiseptic, antispasmodic, aphrodisiac, carminative, digestive, emmenagogue, gastric secretory stimulant, larvicidal, orexigenic, prostaglandin inhibitor, stimulant. **COMPATIBILITIES** Oakmoss, lavandin, bay leaf, Peru balsam, orange, geranium, clary sage, rosemary, lime, petitgrain, mandarin, spice oils.

SAFETY DATA
Nutmeg and mace are generally nontoxic, nonirritant and nonsensitizing. However, used in large doses they show signs of toxicity such as nausea, stupor, and tachycardia, believed to be due to the myristicin content

MYROCARPUS FASTIGIATUS

Cabreuva

FAMILY: FABACEAE (LEGUMINOSAE)

Herbal/Folk Tradition

The wood is highly appreciated for carving and furniture-making. It is used locally to heal wounds, ulcers, and to obviate scars. It was listed in old European pharmacopoeias for its antiseptic qualities.

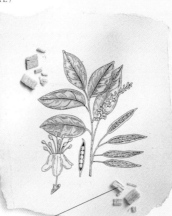

CABREUVA WOOD CHIPPINGS

A graceful, tall tropical tree, 39–49ft (12–15m) high, with a very hard wood, extremely resistant to moisture and mold growth. It yields a balsam when the trunk is damaged, like many other South American trees.

DATAFILE
AROMATHERAPY/ HOME USE **Skin Care:** *Cuts, scars, wounds.* **Respiratory System:** *Chills, coughs.* **Immune System:** *Colds.* **EXTRACTION** Essential oil by steam distillation from wood chippings. **ACTIONS** Antiseptic, balsamic, cicatrizant. **COMPATIBILITIES** It blends well with rose, cassie, mimosa, cedarwood, and rich woody and oriental bases.

SAFETY DATA
Nontoxic, nonirritant, nonsensitizing

MYROXYLON BALSAMUM VAR. BALSAMUM

Tolu balsam

FAMILY: FABACEAE (LEGUMINOSAE)

Herbal/Folk Tradition

It works primarily on the respiratory mucous membranes and is good for non-inflammatory chest complaints, chronic catarrh, croup, and laryngitis. It is used in cough syrups and lozenges.

TOLU BALSAM

A tall tropical tree, similar in appearance to the Peru balsam tree. The balsam is obtained by making V-shaped incisions into the bark and sap wood, often after the trunk has been beaten and scorched. It is a "true" balsam.

DATAFILE

AROMATHERAPY/ HOME USE

Skin Care: *Dry, chapped and cracked skin, eczema, rashes, scabies, sores, wounds.*

Respiratory System: *Bronchitis, catarrh, coughs, croup, laryngitis. "Use as an inhalant by putting about a teaspoon into a steam bath."²²*

EXTRACTION

The crude balsam is collected from the trees. It appears first in liquid form, then solidifies into a brittle mass. An essential oil is obtained from the crude by steam or dry distillation.

ACTIONS

Antitussive, antiseptic, balsamic, expectorant, stimulant.

COMPATIBILITIES

It blends well with mimosa, ylang ylang, sandalwood, labdanum, orange blossom, patchouli, cedarwood, and oriental, spicy, and floral bases.

SAFETY DATA

Available information indicates it to be nontoxic, nonirritant, possible sensitization; see Peru balsam (below)

MYROXYLON BALSAMUM VAR. PEREIRAE

Peru balsam

FAMILY: FABACEAE (LEGUMINOSAE)

Herbal/Folk Tradition

It stimulates the heart, increases blood pressure, and lessens mucous secretions, and is useful for respiratory disorders such as asthma, chronic coughs, and bronchitis.

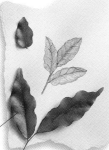

PERU BALSAM LEAVES

A large tropical tree up to 82ft (25m) high, with a straight smooth trunk, beautiful foliage, and fragrant flowers. Every part of the tree contains a resinous juice. Balsam is obtained from the exposed wood after the bark has been stripped.

DATAFILE

AROMATHERAPY/ HOME USE

The balsam (not the oil) is a common contact allergen, which may cause dermatitis. Those who have this sensitivity may also react to benzoin resinoid ("cross-sensitization").

Skin Care: *Dry and chapped skin, eczema, rashes, sores, and wounds.*

Circulation, Muscles, and Joints: *Low blood pressure, rheumatism.*

Respiratory System: *Asthma, bronchitis, coughs.*

Immune System: *Colds.*

Nervous System: *Nervous tension, stress.*

EXTRACTION

Resin-free essential oil is produced from crude balsam by high vacuum dry distillation. (A wood oil, which is considered of inferior quality, is produced by steam distillation from wood chippings.)

ACTIONS

Anti-inflammatory, antiseptic, balsamic, expectorant, parasiticide, stimulant; promotes the growth of epithelial cells.

COMPATIBILITIES

It blends well with ylang ylang, patchouli, petitgrain, sandalwood, rose, spices, and floral and oriental bases.

SAFETY DATA

Nontoxic, nonirritant

MYRTUS COMMUNIS

Myrtle

FAMILY: MYRTACEAE

Herbal/Folk Tradition

The leaves and berries were traditionally thought to be good for diarrhea, dysentery, and catarrh. The leaves and flowers were a major ingredient of "angel's water", a sixteenth-century skin-care lotion.

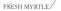

FRESH MYRTLE

A large, fragrant bush or small tree with many tough but slender branches, a brownish-red bark, and small pointed leaves. It has white flowers followed by small black berries.

AROMATHERAPY/ HOME USE

Skin Care: *Acne, hemorrhoids, oily skin, open pores.*
Respiratory System: *Asthma, bronchitis, catarrhal conditions, chronic coughs, tuberculosis – it is a suitable oil to use for children's coughs and chest complaints.*
Immune System: *Colds, flu, infectious disease.*

EXTRACTION

Essential oil by steam distillation from the leaves and twigs, and sometimes the flowers.

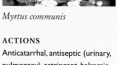

Myrtus communis

ACTIONS

Anticatarrhal, antiseptic (urinary, pulmonary), astringent, balsamic, bactericidal, expectorant, regulator, slightly sedative.

COMPATIBILITIES

Bergamot, lavandin, lavender, clary sage, rosemary, hyssop, bay leaf, lime, laurel, ginger, and spice oils.

SAFETY DATA
Nontoxic, nonirritant, nonsensitizing

NARCISSUS POETICUS

Narcissus

FAMILY: AMARYLLIDACEAE

Herbal/Folk Tradition

The name derives from its narcotic properties; the Greek *narkao* means "to be numb". In France the flowers were used at one time for their antispasmodic properties, said to be useful in hysteria and epilepsy.

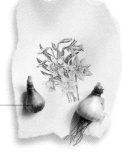

NARCISSUS BULB

A familiar garden flower up to 20in (50cm) high, with long sword-shaped leaves and very fragrant white flowers, having a short yellow trumpet and crisped red edge.

AROMATHERAPY/ HOME USE

Perfume. The bulbs of N. poeticus are more dangerous than those of the daffodil, since they have powerful emetic and irritant qualities. If the flowers are present in any quantity in a closed room, they will produce headache and even vomiting in some people.

EXTRACTION

A concrete and absolute by solvent extraction from the flowers.

ACTIONS

Antispasmodic, aphrodisiac, emetic, narcotic, sedative.

COMPATIBILITIES

It blends well with clove bud, jasmine, neroli, ylang ylang, rose, mimosa, sandalwood, oriental and floral fragrances.

SAFETY DATA
All members of the Amaryllidaceae family, especially the bulbs, have a profound effect on the nervous system, causing paralysis and even, in some cases, death

NARDOSTACHYS JATAMANSI

Spikenard

FAMILY: VALERIANANCEAE

Herbal/Folk Tradition

Spikenard is one of the early aromatics used by the ancient Egyptians and is mentioned in the *Song of Solomon* in the Bible.

The herb was considered good for nausea, flatulent indigestion, menstrual problems, inflammations, and conjunctivitis.

DRIED SPIKENARD ROOT

A tender aromatic herb with a pungent rhizome root.

DATAFILE

AROMATHERAPY/ HOME USE

Skin Care: *Allergies, inflammation, mature skin (rejuvenating), rashes, etc.*

Nervous System: *Insomnia, nervous indigestion, migraine, stress, and tension.*

EXTRACTION

Essential oil by steam distillation from the dried and crushed rhizome and roots.

ACTIONS

Anti-inflammatory, antipyretic, bactericidal, deodorant, fungicidal, laxative, sedative, tonic.

COMPATIBILITIES

It blends well with labdanum, lavender, oakmoss, patchouli, pine needle, vetiver, and spice oils.

SAFETY DATA

Probably similar to Valerian, see page 134, i.e. nontoxic, nonirritant, nonsensitizing

---

OCIMUM BASILICUM

Exotic basil

FAMILY: LAMIACEAE (LABIATAE)

Herbal/Folk Tradition

A popular culinary herb, especially in Italy and France. In the West it is considered a cooling herb and is used for rheumatic pain, irritable skin conditions, and for those of a nervous disposition. It is also widely used in Far Eastern medicine.

LEAVES

FRESH BASIL FLOWERS

Botanically classified as identical with French basil, though it is a larger plant with a harsher odor and different constituents.

DATAFILE

AROMATHERAPY/ HOME USE

None.

Exotic basil is produced mainly in the Comoran Islands. It has a high methyl chavicol content, which is sufficient reason to discard it for therapeutic usage in favor of the French type.

EXTRACTION

Essential oil by steam distillation from the leaves and flowering tops.

ACTIONS

Antidepressant, antiseptic, antispasmodic, carminative,

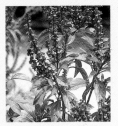

Ocimum basilicum

cephalic, digestive, emmenagogue, expectorant, febrifuge, galactagogue, nervine, prophlyactic, restorative, stimulant of adrenal cortex, stomachic, tonic.

SAFETY DATA

Methyl chavicol is moderately toxic, irritating to the skin, and may be carcinogenic. Basil should be avoided during pregnancy

OCIMUM BASILICUM

French basil

FAMILY: LAMIACEAE (LABIATAE)

Herbal/Folk Tradition

See Exotic basil, page 109.

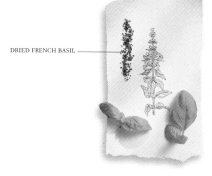

DRIED FRENCH BASIL

A tender, aromatic annual herb, with very dark green, ovate leaves, grayish-green beneath, an erect square stem up to 24in (60cm) high, bearing whorls of two-lipped greenish or pinky-white flowers.

ORIGANUM MARJORANA

Sweet marjoram

FAMILY: LAMIACEAE (LABIATAE)

Herbal/Folk Tradition

A traditional culinary herb and folk remedy. It is a versatile herb, and is fortifying, soothing, and warming; it aids digestive and menstrual problems, and nervous and respiratory complaints.

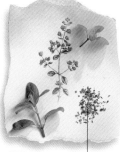

DRIED SWEET MARJORAM

A tender bushy perennial plant (cultivated as an annual in colder climates), up to 24in (60cm) high with a hairy stem, dark green oval leaves, and small grayish-white flowers in clusters or "knots". The whole plant is strongly aromatic.

ORIGANUM VULGARE

Common oregano

FAMILY: LAMIACEAE (LABIATAE)

Herbal/Folk Tradition

A herb of very ancient medical repute. Traditionally used for digestive upsets, respiratory problems (asthma, bronchitis, coughs, etc.), colds, and flu, as well as for inflammations of the mouth and throat.

DRIED HERB

A hardy, bushy, perennial herb up to 35in (90cm) high with an erect hairy stem, dark green ovate leaves, and pinky-purple flowers. A common garden plant with a strong aroma when the leaves are bruised.

DATAFILE

AROMATHERAPY/ HOME USE
None. Do not use on the skin.

EXTRACTION
Essential oil by steam distillation from the dried flowering herb.

ACTIONS
Analgesic, anthelmintic, anti-rheumatic, antiseptic, anti-spasmodic, antitoxic, antiviral, bactericidal, carminative, choleretic, cytoplyactic, diaphoretic, diuretic, emmenagogue, expectorant, febrifuge, fungicidal, parasiticide, rubefacient, stimulant, tonic.

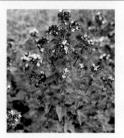

Origanum vulgare

COMPATIBILITIES
It blends well with lavandin, oakmoss, pine, spike lavender, citronella, rosemary, camphor, and cedarwood.

SAFETY DATA
Dermal toxin, skin irritant, mucous membrane irritant. Avoid during pregnancy

---

ORMENIS MULTICAULIS

Maroc chamomile

FAMILY: ASTERACEAE (COMPOSITAE)

Herbal/Folk Tradition

This is one of the more recent oils to appear on the market, and as such it does not have a long history of usage. The oil is distinctly different from the German or the Roman chamomile oils, and is not a replacement.

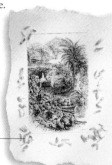

DRIED MAROC CHAMOMILE

A handsome plant, 35–49in (90–125cm) high, with very hairy leaves and tubular yellow flowers, surrounded by white ligulets.

DATAFILE

AROMATHERAPY/ HOME USE
Little is known about its therapeutic history and usage. It has been recommended for sensitive skin, colic, colitis, headache, insomnia, irritability, migraine, amenorrhea, menopause, liver and spleen congestion.

EXTRACTION
Essential oil by steam distillation from the flowering tops.

ACTIONS
Antispasmodic, cholagogue, emmenagogue, hepatic, sedative.

COMPATIBILITIES
It blends well with cypress, lavender, lavandin, vetiver, cedarwood, oakmoss, labdanum, olibanum, and artemisia oils.

SAFETY DATA
Generally nontoxic and nonirritant – more specific safety data is unavailable at present

PELARGONIUM GRAVEOLENS

Geranium

FAMILY: GERANIACEAE

Herbal/Folk Tradition

The British plant herb *Geranium robertanium* and the American *G. maculatum* are the most widely used types in herbal medicine today. They are used for conditions such as dysentery and hemorrhoids.

FRESH LEAVES

A perennial hairy shrub up to 3ft (1m) high with pointed leaves, serrated at the edges, and small pink flowers. The whole plant is aromatic.

DATAFILE

AROMATHERAPY/HOME USE

Skin Care: *Acne, bruises, burns, congested skin, cuts, dermatitis, eczema, hemorrhoids, lice, mature skin, mosquito repellent, oily skin, ringworm, ulcers, wounds.*

Circulation, Muscles, and Joints: *Cellulitis, breast engorgement, edema, poor circulation.*

Respiratory System: *Sore throat, tonsillitis.*

Genitourinary and Endocrine Systems: *Adrenocortical glands and menopausal problems, PMS.*

Nervous System: *Tension, neuralgia, and stress.*

EXTRACTION

Essential oil by steam distillation from leaves, stalks, and flowers.

ACTIONS

Antidepressant, antihemorrhagic, antiflammatory, antiseptic, astringent, cicatrizant, deodorant, diuretic, fungicidal, hemostatic, stimulant (adrenal cortex), styptic, tonic, vermifuge, vulnerary.

COMPATIBILITIES

Lavender, patchouli, clove, rose, orange blossom, sandalwood, jasmine, juniper, bergamot, and other citrus oils.

SAFETY DATA
Nontoxic, nonirritant, generally nonsensitizing; possibly contact dermatitis in hypersensitive individuals, especially with the Bourbon type

---

PETROSELINUM SATIVUM

Parsley

FAMILY: APIACEAE (UMBELLIFERAE)

Herbal/Folk Tradition

Used extensively as a culinary herb, it is a very nutritious plant, high in vitamins A and C. The herb and seed are used medicinally, principally for kidney and bladder problems.

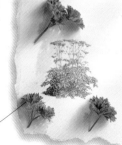

FRESH PARSLEY

A biennial or short-lived perennial herb up to 28in (70cm) high with crinkly bright green foliage, small greenish-yellow flowers, and producing small brown seeds.

DATAFILE

AROMATHERAPY/HOME USE

Circulation, Muscles, and Joints: *Accumulation of toxins, arthritis, broken blood vessels, cellulites, rheumatism, sciatica.*

Digestive System: *Colic, flatulence, indigestion, hemorrhoids.*

Genitourinary System: *Amenorrhea, dysmenorrhea, to aid labor, cystitis, urinary infection.*

EXTRACTION

Essential oil by steam distillation from the seed and the herb. An essential oil is occasionally extracted from the roots, and an oleoresin is also produced by solvent extraction from the seeds.

ACTIONS

Antimicrobial, antirheumatic, antiseptic, astringent, carminative, diuretic, depurative, emmenagogue, febrifuge, hypotensive, laxative, stimulant (mild), stomachic, tonic (uterine).

COMPATIBILITIES

It blends well with rose, orange blossom, cananga, tea tree, oakmoss, clary sage, and spice oils.

SAFETY DATA
Both oils are moderately toxic and irritant, otherwise nonsensitizing. Use in moderation. Avoid during pregnancy

PEUMUS BOLDUS

Boldo leaf

FAMILY: MONIMIACEAE

Herbal/Folk Tradition

In South America it has long been recognized as a valuable cure for gonorrhea. In Western herbalism, the dried leaves are used for genitourinary inflammation, gallstones, liver or gall bladder pain, cystitis, and rheumatism.

DRIED BOLDO LEAF

An evergreen shrub or small tree up to 20ft (6m) high, with slender branches, sessile coarse leaves, and bearing yellowish-green fruit; dried the leaves turn a deep reddish-brown color. The whole plant is aromatic.

DATAFILE

AROMATHERAPY/ HOME USE
None. The oil has powerful therapeutic effects and should be considered harmful to the human organism even in very small doses It should not be used in therapy, either internally or externally.

EXTRACTION
Essential oil by steam distillation of the leaves.

ACTIONS
Antiseptic, cholagogue, diaphoretic, diuretic, hepatic, sedative, tonic, urinary demulcent.

Peumus boldus Native to Chile, naturalized in the Mediterranean region. Some essential oil is produced in Nepal and Vietnam.

SAFETY DATA
Extremely toxic

PILOCARPUS JABORANDI

Jaborandi

FAMILY: RUTACEAE

Herbal/Folk Tradition

Jaborandi induces salivation and most gland secretions; it was also used at one time to promote hair growth. It is considered useful in psoriasis, prurigo, deafness, chronic catarrh, tonsillitis, and particularly dropsy.

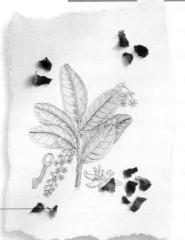

DRIED JABORANDI FLOWERS

A woody shrub up to 6ft (2m) high with a smooth, grayish bark, large brownish-green leathery leaves containing big oil glands, and reddish-purple flowers.

DATAFILE

AROMATHERAPY/ HOME USE
None. Some hypodermic solutions are prepared from pilocarpine, the main active constituent. It is little used in perfumery or flavor work, because of its extreme toxicity.

EXTRACTION
Essential oil by steam distillation from the dried leaflets.

ACTIONS
Antiseptic, diaphoretic, emmenagogue, galactagogue, stimulant (nerve).

SAFETY DATA
Oral toxin, skin irritant, abortifacient

Allspice

FAMILY: MYRTACEAE

Herbal/Folk Tradition

Used for flatulent indigestion and externally for neuralgic or rheumatic pain. Pimento water helps prevent griping pains and is used as a vehicle for medicines that ease dyspepsia and constipation.

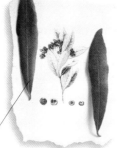

FRESH
ALLSPICE LEAF

An evergreen tree up to 33ft (10m) high. It produces fruit in its third year. Each fruit contains two kidney-shaped green seeds, which turn glossy black when ripe.

DATAFILE

AROMATHERAPY/ HOME USE

Circulation, Muscles, and Joints: *Arthritis, fatigue, muscle cramp, rheumatism, stiffness, etc. Can be used in tiny amounts in a massage oil for chest infections, severe muscle spasm, or extreme cold.*
Respiratory System: *Chills, congested coughs, bronchitis.*
Digestive System: *Cramp, flatulence, indigestion, nausea.*
Nervous System: *Depression, nervous exhaustion, neuralgia, tension, and stress.*

EXTRACTION
Essential oil by steam distillation from the leaves or the fruit. An oleoresin from the berries is also produced.

ACTIONS
Anesthetic, analgesic, antioxidant, antiseptic, carminative, muscle relaxant, rubefacient, stimulant, tonic.

COMPATIBILITIES
It blends well with ginger, geranium, lavender, opopanax, labdanum, ylang ylang, patchouli, orange blossom, oriental and spicy bases.

SAFETY DATA
Contains eugenol, which irritates the mucous membranes, and has been found to cause dermal irritation. Pimenta leaf and berry oil should therefore be used with care in low dilutions only

West Indian bay

FAMILY: MYRTACEAE

Herbal/Folk Tradition

The West Indian bay tree is often grown together with the allspice or pimento bush, then the fruits of both are dried and powdered to make household allspice. The bay leaves are distilled in rum to make the famous old hair tonic.

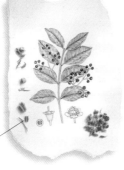

DRIED WEST
INDIAN BAY BARK

A wild-growing tropical evergreen tree up to 26ft (8m) high, with large leathery leaves and aromatic fruits.

DATAFILE

AROMATHERAPY/ HOME USE

Skin Care: *Scalp stimulant, hair rinse for dandruff, greasy, lifeless hair, and promoting growth.*
Circulation, Muscles, and Joints: *Muscular and articular aches and pains, neuralgia, poor circulation, rheumatism, sprains, strains.*
Immune System: *Colds, flu, infectious diseases.*

EXTRACTION
Essential oil by water or steam distillation from the leaves. An oleoresin is also produced in small quantities.

ACTIONS
Analgesic, anticonvulsant, antineuralgic, expectorant, antirheumatic, antiseptic, astringent, stimulant, tonic (for hair).

COMPATIBILITIES
It blends well with lavender, lavandin, rosemary, geranium, ylang ylang, citrus and spice oils.

SAFETY DATA
Moderately toxic due to high eugenol content; a mucous membrane irritant, so use in moderation. Unlike bay laurel, however, it does not appear to cause dermal irritation or sensitization

PIMPINELLA ANISUM

Aniseed

FAMILY: APIACEAE (UMBELLIFERAE)

Herbal/Folk Tradition

Widely used as a domestic spice. The volatile oil content provides the basis for its medicinal applications: dry irritable coughs, bronchitis, and whooping cough. Aniseed tea is used for infant catarrh, also flatulence, colic, and griping pains, painful periods and to promote breast milk.

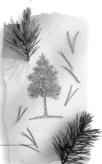

ANISEED SEEDS

An annual herb, less than 3ft (1m) high, with delicate leaves and white flowers.

DATAFILE

AROMATHERAPY/ HOME USE
See Star anise, page 90.

EXTRACTION
Essential oil by steam distillation from the seeds.

ACTIONS
Antiseptic, antispasmodic, carminative, diuretic, expectorant, galactagogue, stimulant, stomachic.

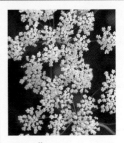

Pimpinella anisum
Native to Greece and Egypt, now widely cultivated. In Turkey, a popular alcholoic drink, raki, is made from the seed.

SAFETY DATA
Contains anethole, which is known to cause dermatitis – avoid in allergic and inflammatory skin conditions. In large doses it is narcotic and slows down the circulation; can lead to cerebral disorders. Use in moderation. Avoid during pregnancy

---

PINUS MUGO VAR. PUMILIO

Dwarf pine

FAMILY: PINACEAE

Herbal/Folk Tradition

A preparation made from the needles has been used internally for bladder, kidney, and rheumatic complaints, as a liniment for rheumatism and muscular pain, and as an inhalant for bronchitis, catarrh, colds, etc.

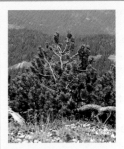

DWARF PINE NEEDLES

A pyramidal shrub or small tree up to 39ft (12m) high with a black bark, stiff and twisted needles borne in clusters, and brown cones, initially of a bluish hue.

DATAFILE

AROMATHERAPY/ HOME USE
None. It is best avoided therapeutically due to irritant hazards.

EXTRACTION
Essential oil by steam distillation from the needles and twigs.

ACTIONS
Analgesic, antimicrobial, antiseptic, antitussive, antiviral, balsamic, diuretic, expectorant, rubefacient.

COMPATIBILITIES
Its unique delicate odor blends well with cedarwood, lavandin,

Pinus mugo var. pumilio
Native to the mountainous regions of central and southern Europe.

rosemary, sage, cananga, labdanum, juniper, and other coniferous oils.

SAFETY DATA
Dermal irritant, common sensitizing agent; otherwise nontoxic

Longleaf pine

FAMILY: PINACEAE

Herbal/Folk Tradition

Pine sawdust has been used for centuries as a highly esteemed household remedy for a variety of ailments. It was valued as a powerful external antiseptic remedy, applied as a poultice.

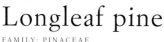

FRESH PINE NEEDLES

STEM WITH BARK

A tall evergreen tree with long needles and a straight trunk, grown for lumber. It exudes an oleoresin from the trunk, and is the largest turpentine source in the United States.

AROMATHERAPY/ HOME USE
Circulation, Muscles, and Joints: *Arthritis, debility, lumbago, muscular aches and pains, poor circulation, rheumatism, stiffness, etc.* Respiratory System: *Asthma, bronchitis, catarrh, sinusitis.*

EXTRACTION
The crude oil is obtained by steam distillation from the sawdust and wood chips from the heartwood and roots of the tree, and then submitted to fractional distillation under atmospheric pressure to produce pine essential oil.

ACTIONS
Analgesic (mild), antirheumatic, antiseptic, bactericidal, expectorant, insecticidal, stimulant.

COMPATIBILITIES
It blends well with rosemary, pine needle, cedarwood, citronella, rosewood, ho leaf, and oakmoss.

SAFETY DATA
Nontoxic, nonirritant (except in concentration), possible sensitization in some individuals

---

Turpentine

FAMILY: PINACEAE

Herbal/Folk Tradition

Known since ancient times for its application to genitourinary and pulmonary infections, digestive complaints, and externally for rheumatic or neuralgic pain and skin conditions.

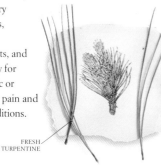

FRESH TURPENTINE

"Gum turpentine" is a term applied to the oleoresin formed as a physiological product in the trunks of various Pinus, Picea, and Abies species. Turpentine refers both to the crude oleoresin and to the distilled and rectified essential oils.

AROMATHERAPY/ HOME USE
See Mastic, page 118.

EXTRACTION
Essential oil by steam (or water) distillation from the crude oleoresin, then rectified.

ACTIONS
Analgesic, antimicrobial, antirheumatic, antiseptic, antispasmodic, balsamic, diuretic, cicatrizant, counterirritant, expectorant, hemostatic, parasiticide, rubefacient, stimulant, tonic, vermifuge.

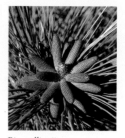

Pinus elliottii
Produced all over the world, and widely used in ointments for aches and pains and in cough and cold remedies.

SAFETY DATA
Enviromental hazard – marine pollutant. Relatively nontoxic and nonirritant; possible sensitization in some individuals. Avoid therapeutic use or employ in moderation only

PINUS SYLVESTRIS

Scotch pine

FAMILY: PINACEAE

Herbal/Folk Tradition

It was used by the Native Americans to prevent scurvy, and to stuff mattresses to repel lice and fleas. As an inhalation it helps relieve bronchial catarrh, asthma, blocked sinuses. The pine kernels are an excellent restorative.

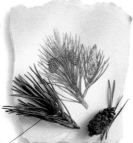

FRESH NEEDLES

SCOTCH PINE CONE

A tall evergreen tree, up to 131ft (40m) high with a flat crown. It has a reddish-brown, deeply fissured bark, long stiff needles that grow in pairs, and pointed brown cones.

DATAFILE

AROMATHERAPY/HOME USE

Skin Care: *Cuts, lice, excessive perspiration, scabies, sores.*
Circulation, Muscles, and Joints: *Arthritis, gout, muscular aches and pains, poor circulation, rheumatism.*
Respiratory System: *Asthma, bronchitis, catarrh, coughs, sinusitis.*
Genitourinary System: *Cystitis, urinary infection.*
Immune System: *Colds, flu.*
Nervous System: *Fatigue, nervous exhaustion, neuralgia.*

EXTRACTION
Essential oil by dry distillation of the needles.

ACTIONS
Antimicrobial, antineuralgic, antirheumatic, antiscorbutic, antiseptic (pulmonary, urinary, hepatic), antiviral, bactericidal, balsamic, cholagogue, choleretic, deodorant, diuretic, expectorant, hypertensive, insecticidal, restorative, rubefacient, stimulant (adrenal cortex, circulatory, nervous), vermifuge.

COMPATIBILITIES
It blends well with cedarwood, rosemary, tea tree, sage, lavender, juniper, lemon, niaouli, eucalyptus, and marjoram.

SAFETY DATA
Nontoxic, nonirritant (except in concentration), possible sensitization. Avoid in allergic skin conditions

---

PIPER CUBEBA

Cubeb

FAMILY: PIPERACEAE

Herbal/Folk Tradition

It has been traditionally used for treating genito-urinary infections, such as gonorrhea, cystitis, urethritis, abscess of the prostate gland, and leucorrhea. It is also used for digestive upsets and respiratory problems.

DRIED CUBEB SEED

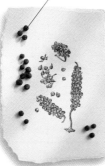

An evergreen climbing vine up to 20ft (6m) high with heart-shaped leaves. Altogether similar to the black pepper plant, except that the fruit or seeds of the cubeb retain their peduncle or stem – thus the name, tailed pepper.

DATAFILE

AROMATHERAPY/HOME USE

Respiratory System: *Bronchitis, catarrh, congestion, chronic coughs, sinusitis, throat infections.*
Digestive System: *Flatulence, indigestion, piles, sluggish digestion.*
Genitourinary System: *Cystitis, leucorrhea, urethritis.*

EXTRACTION
Essential oil by steam distillation from the unripe but fully grown fruits or berries. An oleoresin is also produced in small quantities.

ACTIONS
Antiseptic (pulmonary, genito-urinary), antispasmodic, antiviral, bactericidal, carminative, diuretic, expectorant, stimulant.

COMPATIBILITIES
It blends well with cananga, galbanum, lavender, rosemary, black pepper, allspice, and other spices.

SAFETY DATA
Nontoxic, nonirritant, nonsensitizing. Frequently subject to adulteration

PIPER NIGRUM

Black pepper

FAMILY: PIPERACEAE

Herbal/Folk Tradition

Both black and white pepper have been used in the East for over 4,000 years for medicinal and culinary purposes. In China, white pepper is used to treat malaria, cholera, dysentery, diarrhea, stomach-ache, and other digestive problems.

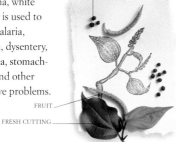

DRIED PEPPERCORN

FRUIT

FRESH CUTTING

A perennial woody vine up to 16ft (5m) high with heart-shaped leaves and white flowers. Berries mature from red to black – black pepper is the fully grown, unripe fruit.

DATAFILE

AROMATHERAPY/ HOME USE
Not compatible with homeopathic treatment.
Skin Care: *Chilblains.*
Circulation, Muscles, and Joints: *Anemia, arthritis, muscular aches and pains, neuralgia, poor circulation, poor muscle tone (muscular atonia), rheumatic pain, sprains, stiffness.*
Respiratory System: *Catarrh, chills.*
Digestive System: *Colic, constipation, diarrhea, flatulence, heartburn, loss of appetite, nausea.*
Immune System: *Colds, flu, infections, and viruses.*

EXTRACTION
Essential oil by steam distillation from dried black peppercorns.

ACTIONS
Analgesic, antimicrobial, antiseptic, antispasmodic, antitoxic, aperitif, aphrodisiac, bactericidal, carminative, diaphoretic, digestive, diuretic, febrifuge, laxative, rubefacient, stimulant (nervous, circulatory, digestive), stomachic, tonic.

COMPATIBILITIES
Frankincense, sandalwood, lavender, rosemary, marjoram, spices, and florals.

SAFETY DATA
Nontoxic, nonsensitizing, irritant in high concentration due to rubefacient properties. Use in moderation only

---

PISTACIA LENTISCUS

Mastic

FAMILY: ANACARDIACEAE

Herbal/Folk Tradition

In the East it is used in the manufacture of confectionery and cordials; it is still used medicinally for diarrhea in children and to sweeten the breath. The oil was used in the West in a similar way to turpentine.

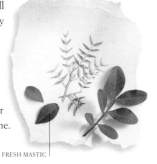

FRESH MASTIC

A small bushy tree or shrub up to 10ft (3m) high, which produces a natural oleoresin from the trunk. Incisions are made in the bark in order to collect the liquid oleoresin, which then hardens into brittle pea-size lumps.

DATAFILE

AROMATHERAPY/ HOME USE
Use with care for:
Skin Care: *Boils, cuts, fleas, insect repellant, lice, ringworm, scabies, wounds.*
Circulation, Muscles, and Joints: *Arthritis, gout, muscular aches and pains, rheumatism, sciatica.*
Respiratory System: *Bronchitis, catarrh, whooping cough.*
Genitourinary System: *Cystitis, leucorrhea, urethritis.*
Immune System: *Colds.*
Nervous System: *Neuralgia.*

EXTRACTION
A resinoid is produced by solvent extraction from the oleoresin, and an essential oil is produced by steam distillation from the oleoresin.

ACTIONS
Antimicrobial, antiseptic, antispasmodic, astringent, diuretic, expectorant, stimulant.

COMPATIBILITIES
Lavender, mimosa, and citrus and floral oils.

SAFETY DATA
Nontoxic, nonirritant, possible sensitization in some individuals

POGOSTEMON CABLIN

Patchouli

FAMILY: LAMIACEAE (LABIATAE)

Herbal/Folk Tradition
The oil is used in the East to scent linen and clothes, and it is believed to help prevent the spread of disease. In China, Japan, and Malaysia the herb is used to treat colds, headaches, nausea, diarrhea, abdominal pain, and halitosis.

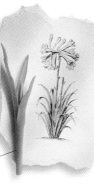

FRESH PATCHOULI

A perennial bushy herb up to 3ft (1m) high with a sturdy, hairy stem, large, fragrant, furry leaves, and white flowers tinged with purple.

DATAFILE

**AROMATHERAPY/
HOME USE**
Skin Care: *Acne, athlete's foot, cracked and chapped skin, dandruff, dermatitis, eczema (weeping), fungal infections, impetigo, insect repellent, oily hair and skin, open pores, sores, wounds, wrinkles.*
Nervous System: *Frigidity, nervous exhaustion, and stress.*

EXTRACTION
Essential oil by steam distillation of the dried leaves.

ACTIONS
Antidepressant, anti-inflammatory, antiemetic, antimicrobial, antiphlogistic, antiseptic, antitoxic, antiviral, aphrodisiac, astringent, bactericidal, carminative, cicatrizant, deodorant, digestive, diuretic, febrifuge, fungicidal, nervine, prophylactic, stimulant (nervous), stomachic, tonic.

COMPATIBILITIES
Labdanum, vetiver, sandalwood, cedarwood, oakmoss, geranium, clove, lavender, rose, orange blossom, cassia, bergamot, myrrh, clary sage, opopanax, and oriental bases.

SAFETY DATA
Nontoxic, nonirritant, nonsensitizing

POLIANTHES TUBEROSA

Tuberose

FAMILY: AGAVACEAE

Herbal/Folk Tradition
The double-flowered variety is grown for ornamental purposes and for use by the cut flower trade. The pure absolute extraction of tuberose is one of the most expensive natural flower oils at the disposal of the modern perfumer.

FRESH
TUBEROSE LEAVES

A tender, tall, slim perennial up to 20in (50cm) high, with long slender leaves, a tuberous root, and large, very fragrant, white lilylike flowers.

DATAFILE

**AROMATHERAPY/
HOME USE**
Used in high-quality perfumes,

EXTRACTION
A concrete and absolute by solvent extraction from the fresh flowers, picked before the petals open. (An essential oil is also obtained by distillation of the concrete.)

ACTIONS
Narcotic.

COMPATIBILITIES
Gardenia, violet, opopanax, rose, jasmine, carnation, orris, Peru balsam, orange blossom, and ylang ylang.

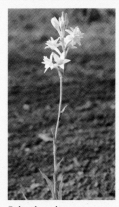

Polianthes tuberosa

SAFETY DATA
No safety data available – often adulterated

PRUNUS DULCIS VAR. AMARA

Bitter almond

FAMILY: ROSACEAE

Herbal/Folk Tradition

A "fixed" oil commonly known as "sweet almond oil" is made by pressing the kernels from both the sweet and bitter almond trees. It is used as a laxative, for bronchitis, heartburn, coughs, and disorders of the kidneys, bladder, and biliary ducts.

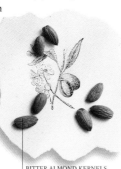

BITTER ALMOND KERNELS

The almond tree grows to a height of about 7m (23ft) and has pinky-white blossom. It is classified as a drupe.

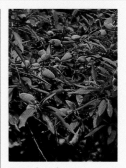

DATAFILE

AROMATHERAPY/ HOME USE
None. It should not be used therapeutically, either internally or externally.

EXTRACTION
Essential oil by steam distillation from the kernels. The nuts are pressed and macerated in warm water for 12–24 hours before the oil is extracted. It is during this process that the prussic acid is formed; it is not present in the raw seed. Most commercial bitter almond oil is rectified to remove all prussic acid.

Bitter almond

ACTIONS
Anesthetic, antispasmodic, narcotic, vermifuge (FFPA).

SAFETY DATA
Prussic acid, also known as hydrocyanic acid or cyanide, is a well-known poison. Benzaldehyde is also moderately toxic

---

ROSA X CENTIFOLIA

Cabbage rose

FAMILY: ROSACEAE

Herbal/Folk Tradition

Up to the Middle Ages the rose was an essential remedy, used for a wide range of disorders, from digestive and menstrual problems to headaches, fever (plague), eye infections, and skin complaints.

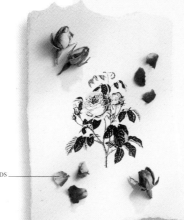

DRIED ROSE BUDS

The rose that is generally used for oil production is strictly a hybrid involving R. x centifolia, R. gallica, *and a few other roses. Known as* rose de mai, *it grows to 8ft (2.5m) high and has a mass of pink or rosy-purple flowers.*

DATAFILE

AROMATHERAPY/ HOME USE
See Damask rose, page 121.

EXTRACTION
See Damask rose, page 121.

ACTIONS
See Damask rose, page 121.

COMPATIBILITIES
It blends well with jasmine, cassie, mimosa, orange blossom, geranium, bergamot, lavender, clary sage, sandalwood, guaiacwood, patchouli, benzoin, chamomile, Peru balsam, clove, and palmarosa.

SAFETY DATA
Nontoxic, nonirritant, nonsensitizing

ROSA X DAMASCENA

Damask rose

FAMILY: ROSACEAE

DAMASK ROSE PETALS

Herbal/Folk Tradition

Culpepers's *Complete Herbal* indicates that "oil of roses is used by itself to cool hot inflammations or swellings, and to bind and stay fluxes of humours to sores."[23] Rose hips are still current in the British Herbal Pharmacopoeia, mainly because of their high vitamin C content. See also Cabbage rose, page 120.

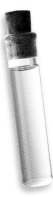

The essential oil is a pale yellow or olive yellow liquid with a very rich, deep, sweet-floral, slightly spicy scent.

Small prickly shrub between 3–6ft (1–2m) high, with pink fragrant blooms and whitish hairy leaves.

DATAFILE

AROMATHERAPY/ HOME USE

Skin Care: Broken capillaries, conjunctivitis (rose water), dry skin, eczema, herpes, mature and sensitive complexions, wrinkles.

Circulation, Muscles, and Joints: Palpitations, poor circulation.

Respiratory System: Asthma, coughs, hay fever.

Digestive System: Cholecystitis, liver congestion, nausea.

Genitourinary System: Irregular menstruation, leucorrhea, menorrhagia, uterine disorders.

Nervous System: Depression, impotence, insomnia, frigidity, headache, nervous tension, and stress-related complaints. The

rose, traditionally associated with Venus, the goddess of love and beauty, induces a feeling of well-being and happiness.

EXTRACTION

Essential oil by water or steam distillation from the fresh petals. Rose water is produced as a by-product of this process. Concrete and absolute by solvent extraction from the fresh petals. A rose leaf absolute is also produced in small quantities in France.

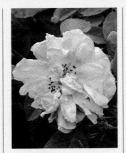

Damask rose

ACTIONS

Antidepressant, antiphlogistic, antiseptic, antispasmodic, anti-tubercular agent, antiviral, aphrodisiac, astringent,

bactericidal, choleretic, cicatrizant, depurative, emmenagogue, hemostatic, hepatic, laxative, regulator of appetite, sedative (nervous), stomachic, tonic (heart, liver, stomach, uterus).

COMPATIBILITIES

It blends well with most oils and is useful for "rounding off" blends. The Bulgarian type is considered superior in perfumery work.

SAFETY DATA

Nontoxic, nonirritant, nonsensitizing

Rosemary

FAMILY: LAMIACEAE (LABIATAE)

FRESH ROSEMARY

Herbal/Folk Tradition

One of the earliest plants to be used for food, medicine, and magic. Sprigs of rosemary were burned at shrines in ancient Greece, fumigations were used in the Middle Ages to drive away evil spirits and as a protection against plague.

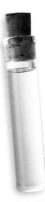

It has been used for a wide range of complaints including respiratory and circulatory disorders, liver congestion, digestive and nervous complaints, muscular and rheumatic pain, skin and hair problems. It is current in the *British Herbal Pharmacopoeia* as a specific for "depressive states with general debility and indications of cardiovascular weakness".[24]

A shrubby evergreen bush up to 6ft (2m) high, with silvery-green, needle-shaped leaves and pale blue flowers. The whole plant is strongly aromatic.

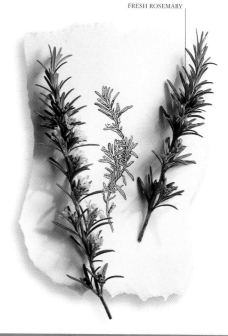

DATAFILE

AROMATHERAPY HOME USE

Skin Care: *Acne, dandruff, dermatitis, eczema, greasy hair, insect repellent, lice, promotes hair growth, regulates seborrhea, scabies, stimulates scalp, varicose veins.*
Circulation, Muscles, and Joints: *Arteriosclerosis, fluid retention, gout, muscular pain, palpitations, poor circulation, rheumatism.*
Respiratory System: *Asthma, bronchitis, whooping cough.*
Digestive System: *Colitis, dyspepsia, flatulence, hepatic disorders, hypercholesterolemia, jaundice.*

Genitourinary System: *Dysmenorrhea, leucorrhea.*
Immune System: *Colds, flu, infections.*
Nervous System: *Debility, headaches, hypotension, neuralgia, mental fatigue, nervous exhaustion, and stress-related disorders.*

EXTRACTION

Essential oil by steam distillation of the fresh flowering tops or (in Spain) the whole plant (poorer quality).

ACTIONS

Analgesic, antimicrobial, antioxidant, antirheumatic, antiseptic, antispasmodic, aphrodisiac, astringent, carminative, cephalic, cholagogue, choleretic, cicatrizant, cordial, cytophylactic, diaphoretic, digestive, diuretic, emmenagogue, fungicidal, hepatic, hypertensive, nervine, parasiticide, restorative, rubefacient, stimulant (circulatory, adrenal cortex, hepatobiliary), stomachic, sudorific, tonic (nervous, general), vulnerary.

COMPATIBILITIES

It blends well with olibanum, lavender, lavandin, citronella, oregano, thyme, pine, basil, peppermint, labdanum, elemi, cedarwood, petitgrain, cinnamon, and other spice oils.

SAFETY DATA

Nontoxic, nonirritant (in dilution only), nonsensitizing. Avoid during pregnancy. Not to be used by epileptics.
Contraindicated in cases of high blood pressure

Rue

FAMILY: RUTACEAE

Herbal/Folk Tradition

A favored remedy of the ancients, especially as an antidote to poison. It was seen as a magic herb by many cultures and as a protection against evil. It was also used for nervous afflictions.

FRESH RUE

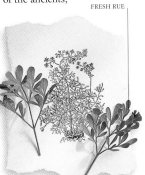

An ornamental, shrubby herb with a strong, aromatic, bitter, or acrid scent. It has tough, woody branches, small, smooth, bluish-green leaves, and greeny-yellow flowers.

DATAFILE

AROMATHERAPY/ HOME USE

None. It should not be used in aromatherapy.

EXTRACTION

Essential oil by steam distillation from the fresh herb.

ACTIONS

Antitoxic, antitussive, antiseptic, antispasmodic, diuretic, emmenagogue, insecticidal, nervine, rubefacient, stimulant, tonic, vermifuge.

Ruta graveolens
Native to the Mediterranean, found growing wild in Spain, Morocco, Corsica, Sardinia, and Algeria.

SAFETY DATA

Oral toxin (due to main constituent). Skin and mucous membrane irritant. Abortifacient. "Rue oil should never be used in perfumery or flavor work."[25]

Spanish sage

FAMILY: LAMIACEAE (LABIATAE)

Herbal/Folk Tradition

In Spain it is regarded as a "cure-all". Believed to promote longevity and protect against infection. Used for rheumatism, digestive complaints, menstrual problems, infertility, and nervous weakness.

SMALL PURPLE FLOWERS

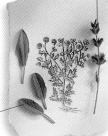

FRESH LEAF

An evergreen shrub, similar to the garden sage but with narrower leaves and small purple flowers. The whole plant is aromatic with a scent reminiscent of spike lavender.

DATAFILE	

AROMATHERAPY/ HOME USE

Skin Care: *Acne, cuts, dandruff, dermatitis, eczema, gingivitis gum infections, hair loss, sores, sweating.*
Circulation, Muscles, and Joints: *Arthritis, debility, fluid retention, muscular aches, poor circulation, rheumatism.*
Respiratory System: *Asthma, coughs, laryngitis.*
Digestive System: *Jaundice, liver congestion.*
Genitourinary System: *Amenorrhea, dysmenorrhea,*
Immune System: *Colds, flu.*
Nervous System: *Headaches, nervous exhaustion, and stress.*

EXTRACTION

Essential oil by steam distillation.

ACTIONS

Antidepressant, anti-inflammatory, antimicrobial, antiseptic, antispasmodic, astringent, carminative, deodorant, depurative, digestive, emmenagogue, expectorant, febrifuge, hypotensive, nervine, regulator (of seborrhea), stimulant (hepatobiliary, adrenocortical glands, circulation), stomachic, tonic (nerve and general).

COMPATIBILITIES

Rosemary, lavender, pine, clary sage, citronella, eucalyptus.

SAFETY DATA

Relatively nontoxic, nonirritant, nonsensitizing. Avoid during pregnancy; use in moderation

SALVIA OFFICINALIS

Common sage

FAMILY: LAMIACEAE (LABIATAE)

Herbal/Folk Tradition

A herb of ancient repute, valued as a culinary and medicinal plant. It has been used for disorders including respiratory infections, menstrual difficulties, and digestive complaints. It was believed to strengthen the senses and memory.

FRESH COMMON SAGE

An evergreen, shrubby, perennial herb up to 32in (80cm) high with a woody base, soft, silver, oval leaves, and a mass of deep blue or violet flowers.

DATAFILE

AROMATHERAPY/ HOME USE
None. Use with care or avoid in therapeutic work altogether – Spanish sage or clary sage are good alternatives.

EXTRACTION
Essential oil by steam distillation from the dried leaves. A so-called oleoresin is also produced from the exhausted plant material.

ACTIONS
Anti-inflammatory, antimicrobial, antioxidant, antiseptic, antispasmodic, astringent, digestive, diuretic, emmenagogue, febrifuge, hypertensive, insecticidal, laxative, stomachic, tonic.

COMPATIBILITIES
It blends well with lavandin, rosemary, rosewood, lavender, hyssop, lemon, and other citrus oils.

SAFETY DATA
Oral toxin (due to thujone). Abortifacient; avoid in pregnancy. Avoid in epilepsy. Contraindicated in cases of high blood pressure

---

SALVIA SCLAREA

Clary sage

FAMILY: LAMIACEAE (LABIATAE)

Herbal/Folk Tradition

This herb was highly esteemed in the Middle Ages and was used for digestive disorders, kidney disease, uterine and menstrual complaints, for cleansing ulcers, and as a general nerve tonic.

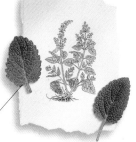

FRESH LEAF

Stout biennial or perennial herb up to 3ft (1m) high with large, hairy leaves, green with a hint of purple, and small blue flowers.

DATAFILE

AROMATHERAPY/ HOME USE
Skin Care: *Acne, boils, dandruff, hair loss, inflammation, oily skin, ophthalmia, ulcers, wrinkles.*
Circulation, Muscles, and Joints: *High blood pressure, muscular aches and pains.*
Respiratory System: *Asthma, throat infections.*
Digestive System: *Cramp, dyspepsia, flatulence.*
Genitourinary System: *Amenorrhea, labor pain, dysmenorrhea, leucorrhea.*
Nervous System: *Depression, frigidity, impotence, migraine, nervous tension, and stress.*

EXTRACTION
Essential oil by steam distillation from flowering tops and leaves.

ACTIONS
Anticonvulsive, antidepressant, antiphlogistic, antiseptic, anti-spasmodic, aphrodisiac, astringent, bactericidal, carminative, cicatrizant, deodorant, digestive, emmenagogue, euphoric, hypotensive, nervine, sedative, stomachic, tonic, uterine.

COMPATIBILITIES
Juniper, lavender, cilantro, pine, cardomon, geranium, sandalwood, jasmine, frankincense, and citrus oils.

SAFETY DATA
Nontoxic, nonirritant, nonsensitizing. Avoid during pregnancy. Do not use clary sage oil while drinking alcohol; it can induce a narcotic effect

SANTALUM ALBUM

Sandalwood

FAMILY: SANTALACEAE

Herbal/Folk Tradition

One of the oldest known perfume materials, used for at least 4,000 years as a cosmetic and perfume all over the East. The Chinese use it to treat stomachache, gonorrhea, choleraic difficulties, and skin complaints.

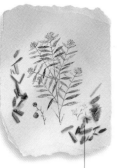

SANDALWOOD CHIPPINGS

A small evergreen, parasitic tree up to 30ft (9m) high with brown-gray trunk and many smooth, slender branches. It has leathery leaves and small pinky-purple flowers.

DATAFILE	
AROMATHERAPY/ HOME USE	**ACTIONS**
Skin Care: *Acne, dry, cracked, and chapped skin, aftershave (barber's rash), greasy skin, moisturizer.*	Antidepressant, antiphlogistic, antiseptic (urinary/pulmonary), antispasmodic, aphrodisiac, astringent, bactericidal, carminative, cicatrizant, diuretic, expectorant, insecticidal, sedative, tonic.
Respiratory System: *Bronchitis, catarrh, dry coughs, laryngitis, sore throat.*	
Digestive System: *Diarrhea, nausea.*	**COMPATIBILITIES**
Genitourinary System: *Cystitis.* **Nervous System:** *Depression, insomnia, nervous tension, and stress-related complaints.*	Rose, violet, tuberose, clove, lavender, black pepper, bergamot, rosewood, mimosa, geranium, labdanum, oakmoss, benzoin, vetiver, patchouli, cassie, costus, myrrh, jasmine.
EXTRACTION Essential oil by water or steam distillation from the roots and heartwood, powdered and dried.	

SAFETY DATA
Nontoxic, nonirritant, nonsensitizing

SANTOLINA CHAMAECYPARISSUS

Santolina

FAMILY: ASTERACEAE (COMPOSITAE)

Herbal/Folk Tradition

It was used as an antidote to all sorts of poison, and to expel worms. It was used to keep away moths from linen, to repel mosquitoes, and as a remedy for insect bits, warts, scabs, and plantar warts (verruccae).

FRESH
SANTOLINA LEAVES

An evergreen, woody shrub with whitish-gray foliage and small, bright yellow, ball-shaped flowers borne on long single stalks. The whole plant has a strong rank odor, a bit like chamomile.

DATAFILE	
AROMATHERAPY/ HOME USE None. No safety data is currently available. It is likely to be highly toxic.	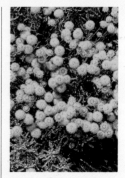
EXTRACTION Essential oil by steam distillation from the seeds.	
ACTIONS Antispasmodic, antitoxic, anthelmintic, insecticidal, stimulant, vermifuge.	

Santolina chamaecyparissus Native to Italy, now common throughout the Mediterranean region. Much grown as a popular border herb.

SAFETY DATA
Oral toxin

SASSAFRAS ALBIDUM

Sassafras

FAMILY: LAURACEAE

Herbal/Folk Tradition

It has been used for treating high blood pressure, rheumatism, arthritis, gout, menstrual and kidney problems, and for skin complaints. The wood and bark yield a bright yellow dye.

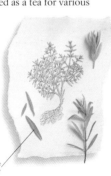

FRESH SASSAFRAS

A deciduous tree up to 131ft (40m) high with many slender branches, a soft and spongy orange-brown bark, and small yellow-green flowers. The bark and wood are aromatic.

DATAFILE

AROMATHERAPY/ HOME USES
None. It should not be used in therapy, either internally or externally.

EXTRACTION
Essential oil by steam distillation from the dried root bark chips.

ACTIONS
Antiviral, diaphoretic, diuretic, carminative, pediculicide (destroys lice), stimulant.

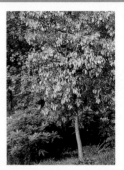

Sassafras albidum
Native to eastern parts of the United States; the oil is produced mainly from Florida to Canada and in Mexico.

SAFETY DATA

Highly toxic – ingestion of even small amounts has been known to cause death. Carcinogen. Irritant. Abortifacient

---

SATUREJA HORTENSIS

Summer savory

FAMILY: LAMIACEAE (LABIATAE)

Herbal/Folk Tradition

A popular culinary herb, with a peppery flavor. It has been used as a tea for various ailments including digestive and respiratory complaints and menstrual disorders. Used externally, the leaves bring relief from insect bites.

FRESH LEAF OF SUMMER SAVORY

An annual herb up to 18in (45cm) high with slender, erect, slightly hairy stems, linear leaves and small, pale lilac flowers.

DATAFILE

AROMATHERAPY/ HOME USE
None. It should not be used on the skin.

EXTRACTION
Essential oil by steam distillation from the whole dried herb. An oleoresin is also produced by solvent extraction.

ACTIONS
Anticatarrhal, antiputrescent, antispasmodic, aphrodisiac, astringent, bactericidal, carminative, cicatrizant, emmenagogue, expectorant, fungicidal, stimulant, vermifuge.

COMPATIBILITIES
It blends well with lavender, lavandin, pine needle, oakmoss, rosemary, and citrus oils.

SAFETY DATA

Dermal toxin, dermal irritant, mucous membrane irritant. Avoid during pregnancy

SATUREJA MONTANA

Winter savory

FAMILY: LAMIACEAE (LABIATAE)

Herbal/Folk Tradition

It has been used as a culinary herb since antiquity, much in the same way as summer savory. It was used as a digestive remedy, especially good for colic, and in Germany it is used particularly for diarrhea.

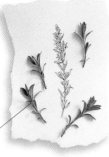

FRESH SPRIG OF WINTER SAVORY

A bushy perennial subshrub up to 16in (40cm) high with woody stems at the base, linear leaves, and pale purple flowers.

DATAFILE

AROMATHERAPY/HOME USE
None. It should not be used on the skin.

EXTRACTION
Essential oil by steam distillation from the whole herb. Oleoresin is produced by solvent extraction.

ACTIONS
Anticatarrhal, antiputrescent, antispasmodic, aphrodisiac, astringent, bactericidal, carminative, cicatrizant, emmenagogue, expectorant, fungicidal, stimulant, vermifuge.

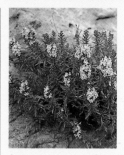

*Satureja montana
Native to the Mediterranean region, now found all over Europe, Russia and Turkey.*

SAFETY DATA
See Summer savory, page 126

SAUSSUREA COSTUS

Costus

FAMILY: ASTERACEA (COMPOSITAE)

Herbal/Folk Tradition

The root has been used for millennia in India and China for digestive complaints, respiratory conditions, as a stimulant, and for infection including typhoid and cholera. It is also used as an incense.

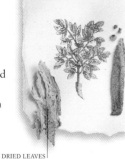

DRIED LEAVES

A large, erect, perennial plant up to 6ft (2m) high with a thick, tapering root and numerous almost black flowers.

DATAFILE

AROMATHERAPY/HOME USE
Costus is not recommended for aromatherapy or home use because it is a common and severe dermal sensitizer. In a recent skin test, it produced sensitization reactions in all 25 volunteers.

EXTRACTION
The dried roots are macerated in warm water, then subjected to steam distillation followed by solvent extraction of the distilled water. (A concrete and absolute are also produced in small quantities.)

ACTIONS
Antiseptic, antispasmodic, antiviral, bactericidal, carminative, digestive, expectorant, febrifuge, hypotensive, stimulant, stomachic, tonic.

COMPATIBILITIES
Patchouli, ylang ylang, opopanax, and oriental and floral fragrances.

SAFETY DATA
Although costus is classified as nontoxic and nonirritant, it is a severe dermal sensitizer

Schinus molle

FAMILY: ANACARDIACEAE

Herbal/Folk Tradition

In Greece and other Mediterranean countries an intoxicating beverage is made from the fruits of the tree. The fruit is used as a substitute for black pepper; this happened during World War II, when black pepper oil was unavailable.

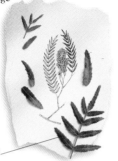

FRESH LEAVES

A tropical evergreen tree up to 65ft (20m) high, with graceful, drooping branches, feathery foliage and fragrant yellow flowers. The berries or fruit have an aromatic, peppery flavor.

DATAFILE	
AROMATHERAPY/ HOME USE Not compatible with homeopathic treatment. **Skin Care:** *Chilblains.* **Circulation, Muscles, and Joints:** *Anemia, arthritis, muscular ache, neuralgia, poor circulation, poor muscle tone, rheumatic pain, stiffness.* **Respiratory System:** *Catarrh, chills.* **Digestive System:** *Appetite loss, colic, constipation, nausea, diarrhea, flatulence, heartburn,* **Immune System:** *Colds, flu, infections, and viruses.*	**EXTRACTION** Essential oil by steam distillation from the fruit or berries. An oil from the leaf is produced in small quantities. **ACTIONS** Antiseptic, antiviral, bactericidal, carminative, stimulant, stomachic. **COMPATIBILITIES** It blends well with oakmoss, clove, nutmeg, cinnamon, black pepper, and eucalyptus.

SAFETY DATA
Nontoxic, nonirritant, nonsensitizing

Spanish broom

FAMILY: FABACEAE (LEGUMINOSAE)

Herbal/Folk Tradition

Spanish broom has similar, but stronger, therapeutic properties to those of common broom, used to treat cardiac dropsy, myocardial weakness, tachycardia, and profuse menstruation.

PEA-LIKE FRAGRANT FLOWERS

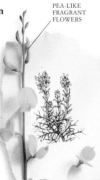

A decorative plant, up to 10ft (3m) high with upright woody branches and tough flexible stems. It has bright green leaves and large, yellow, pealike fragrant flowers, also bearing its seed pods or legumes.

DATAFILE	
AROMATHERAPY/ HOME USE None. In large doses, it causes vomiting, renal irritation, weakens the heart, depresses the nerve cells, and lowers the blood pressure, and in extreme cases causes death. **EXTRACTION** An absolute is obtained by solvent extraction from the dried flowers. **ACTIONS** Antihemorrhagic, cardioactive, diuretic, cathartic, emmenagogue, narcotic, vasoconstrictor.	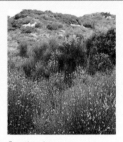 *Spartium junceum* **COMPATIBILITIES** It blends well with rose, tuberose, cassie, mimosa, violet, vetiver, and herbaceous-type fragrances.

SAFETY DATA
Sparteine, contained in the flowers as the main active constituent, is toxic

STYRAX BENZOIN

Benzoin

FAMILY: STYRACACEAE

Herbal/Folk Tradition

Used for thousands of years in the East as a medicine and incense. In the West, best known as the compound tincture friars balsam, used for respiratory complaints. Externally it is used for cuts and irritable skin; used internally to aid digestion.

BENZOIN RESIN

A large tropical tree up to 65ft (20m) high with pale green citruslike leaves, whitish underneath, bearing hard-shelled flattish fruit.

DATAFILE

AROMATHERAPY/HOME USE
Skin Care: *Cuts, chapped skin, inflammations, and irritations.*
Circulation, Muscles, and Joints: *Arthritis, gout, poor circulation, rheumatism.*
Respiratory System: *Asthma, bronchitis, colic, coughs, laryngitis.*
Immune System: *Flu.*
Nervous System: *Nervous tension.*

EXTRACTION
Crude benzoin is collected directly from the trees. Benzoin resinoid is prepared from the crude using solvents.

ACTIONS
Anti-inflammatory, antioxidant, antiseptic, astringent, carminative, cordial, deodorant, diuretic, expectorant, sedative, styptic, vulnerary.

COMPATIBILITIES
Blends well with sandalwood, rose, jasmine, myrrh, cypress, juniper, lemon, cilantro, and other spice oils.

SAFETY DATA
Nontoxic, nonirritant, possible sensitization. Compound benzoin tincture is "regarded as moderately toxic, due probably to occasional contact dermatitis developed in some individuals ... which contains, in addition to benzoin, aloe, storax, Tolu balsam and others."[26]

SYZYGIUM AROMATICUM

Clove

FAMILY: MYRTACEAE

Herbal/Folk Tradition

Used as a domestic spice worldwide. Tincture of cloves has been used for skin infections, digestive upsets, for intestinal parasites; to ease the pain of childbirth, and toothache.

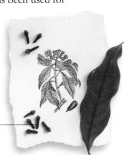

DRIED CLOVES

A slender evergreen tree up to 39ft (12m) high. Its bright green leaves stand in pairs on short stalks. The long buds have a rosy-pink corolla at the tip; as the corolla fades the calyx turns red. These are beaten from the tree and dried.

DATAFILE

AROMATHERAPY/HOME USE
Only use clove bud oil.
Skin Care: *Acne, athlete's foot, bruises, burns, cuts, mosquito repellent, toothache, ulcers.*
Circulation, Muscles, and Joints: *Arthritis, rheumatism, sprains.*
Respiratory System: *Asthma, bronchitis.*
Digestive System: *Colic, nausea.*
Immune System: *Colds, flu,*

EXTRACTION
Essential oil by water distillation from buds or eaves, or by steam distillation from stalks or stems.

ACTIONS
Anthelmintic, antibiotic, anti-aphrodisiac, emetic, antihistaminic, antirheumatic, antineuralgic, anti-oxidant, antiseptic, antiviral, , carminative, counter-irritant, expectorant, larvicidal, stimulant, spasmolytic, stomachic, vermifuge.

COMPATIBILITIES
Rose, lavender, vanillin, clary sage, bergamot, bay leaf, lavandin, allspice, ylang ylang, and cananga.

SAFETY DATA
All clove oil can cause skin and mucous membrane irritation; clove bud and stem oil may cause dermatitis. Clove bud is the least toxic of the tree oils because of the lower eugenol percentage. Use in moderation only, in low dilution (less than 1 per cent)

TAGETES MINUTA

Tagetes

FAMILY: ASTERACEAE (COMPOSITAE)

Herbal/Folk Tradition

In China the flowers of the African marigold are used for whooping cough, colds, colic, mumps, sore eyes, and mastitis. In India flowering tops of French marigold are distilled into a solvent, such as sandalwood oil, to make a perfume.

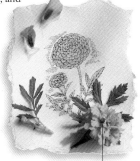

FRESH TAGETES FLOWER

A strongly scented annual herb about 12in (30cm) high with bright orange, daisylike flowers and green oval leaves.

DATAFILE

AROMATHERAPY/ HOME USE

Skin Care: *Bunions, calluses, corns, fungal infections.*

EXTRACTION

An essential oil by steam distillation from the fresh flowering herb. An absolute and concrete by solvent extraction from the fresh flowering herb.

ACTIONS

Anthelmintic, antispasmodic, bactericidal, carminative, diaphoretic, emmenagogue, fungicidal, stomachic.

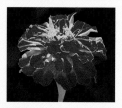

*Tagetes minuta
Native to South America
and Mexico.*

COMPATIBILITIES

It blends well with clary sage, lavender, jasmine, bergamot, and other citrus oils in very small percentages.

SAFETY DATA

"It is quite possible that 'tagetone' (the main constituent) is harmful to the human organism."[27] Some reported cases of dermatitis with the tagetes species. Use with care, in moderation

TANACETUM VULGARE

Tansy

FAMILY: ASTERACEAE (COMPOSITAE)

Herbal/Folk Tradition

FRESH TANSY

It has a long history of medicinal use, especially among gypsies, and is regarded as a "cure-all". It was used to expel worms, to treat colds and fever, prevent miscarriage, and ease dyspepsia.

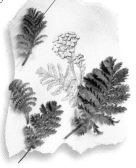

A hardy perennial wayside herb, up to 3ft (1m) high, with a smooth stem, dark ferny leaves, and small, round brilliant yellow flowers borne in clusters. The whole plant is strongly scented.

DATAFILE

AROMATHERAPY/ HOME USE

None. It should not be used in aromatherapy, either internally or externally.

EXTRACTION

Essential oil by steam distillation from the whole herb (aerial parts).

ACTIONS

Anthelmintic, anti-inflammatory, antispasmodic, carminative, diaphoretic, digestive, emmenagogue, febrifuge, nervine, stimulant, tonic, vermifuge.

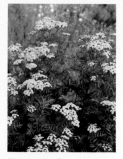

*Tanacetum vulgare
Native to central Europe,
nationalized in North
America, and now found in
most temperate regions of the
world.*

SAFETY DATA

Oral toxin – due to high thujone content. Abortifacient

THUJA OCCIDENTALIS

Thuja

FAMILY: CUPRESSACEAE

Herbal/Folk Tradition

Used as an incense by ancient civilizations.
A decoction of leaves
has been used for
coughs, fever,
intestinal parasites,
venereal diseases,
and cystitis. The
ointment has
been used for
rheumatism, gout,
warts, and plantar
warts (verrucae).

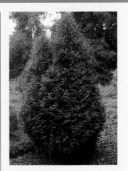

THUJA SEEDS

*A pyramid-shaped coniferous tree up to 65ft (20m) high
with scalelike leaves and broadly winged seeds. The tree
must be fifteen years old before it is used for oil production.*

DATAFILE

**AROMATHERAPY/
HOME USE**
None. It should not be used in
aromatherapy, either internally
or externally.

EXTRACTION
Essential oil by steam distillation
from the leaves, twigs, and bark.

ACTIONS
Antirheumatic, astringent,
diuretic, emmenagogue,
expectorant, insect repellent,
rubefacient, stimulant (nerves,
uterus, and heart muscles),
tonic, vermifuge.

*Thuja occidentalis
Native to northeastern
North America; cultivated
in France. The oil is
produced mainly in Canada
and the United States.*

SAFETY DATA
Oral toxin – poisonous due to high thujone content. Abortifacient

---

THYMUS CAPITATUS

Spanish oregano

FAMILY: LAMIACEAE (LABIATAE)

Herbal/Folk Tradition

The properties and oil of Spanish
oregano (*Thymus
capitatus*) are
similar to the
common thyme
(*T. vulgaris*); it
also shares
many qualities
with common
oregano or wild
marjoram
(*Origanum
vulgare*).

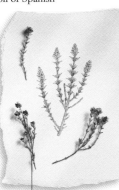

SPANISH OREGANO FLOWERS

*A perennial creeping herb with a woody stem, small dark
green leaves, and pink or white flowers borne in clusters.*

DATAFILE

**AROMATHERAPY/
HOME USE**
None. It should not be used on
the skin.

EXTRACTION
Essential oil by steam distillation
from the dried flowering tops.

ACTIONS
See Common oregano,
page 111.

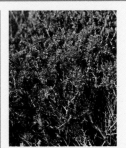

*Thymus capitatus
Native to the Middle East and
Asia Minor; grows wild in
Spain. The oil is produced in
Spain, Israel, Lebanon, Syria,
and Turkey.*

SAFETY DATA
Dermal toxin, skin irritant, mucous membrane irritant

THYMUS VULGARIS

Common thyme

FAMILY: LAMIACEAE (LABIATAE)

Herbal/Folk Tradition

One of the earliest medicinal plants in Western herbal medicine, its main areas of application are respiratory problems, digestive complaints, and the

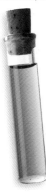

prevention and treatment of infection. In the *British Herbal Pharmacopoeia* it is indicated for dyspepsia, chronic gastritis, bronchitis, pertussis, asthma, children's diarrhea, laryngitis, tonsillitis, and enuresis in children.

FRESH THYME

A perennial evergreen subshrub up to 18in (45cm) high with a woody root and much-branched stem. It has gray-green, aromatic leaves and pale purple or white flowers.

DATAFILE

AROMATHERAPY/ HOME USE
Can irritate mucous membranes, cause dermal irritation and may cause sensitization in some individuals. Use in moderation, in low dilution only. Best avoided during pregnancy.
Skin Care: *Abscess, acne, bruises, burns, cuts, dermatitis, eczema, insect bites, lice, gum infections, oily skin, scabies.*
Circulation, Muscles, and Joints: *Arthritis, cellulitis, gout, muscular aches and pains, obesity, edema, poor circulation, rheumatism,*

sprains, sports injuries.
Respiratory System: *Asthma, bronchitis, catarrh, coughs, laryngitis, sinusitis, sore throat, tonsillitis.*
Digestive System: *Diarrhea, dyspepsia, flatulence.*
Genitourinary System: *Cystitis, urethritis.*
Immune System: *Chills, colds, flu, infectious diseases.*
Nervous System: *Headaches, insomnia, nervous debility, and stress-related complaints.*

EXTRACTION
Essential oil by water or steam distillation from the fresh or partially dried leaves and flowering tops. "Red thyme oil" is the crude distillate. "White thyme oil" is produced by further redistillation or rectification.

ACTIONS
Anthelmintic, antimicrobial, antioxidant, antiputrescent, antirheumatic, antiseptic (intestinal, pulmonary, genitourinary), antispasmodic, antitussive, antitoxic, aperitif,

astringent, aphrodisiac, bactericidal, balsamic, carminative, cicatrizant, diuretic, emmenagogue, nervine, revulsive, rubefacient, parasiticide, stimulant (immune system, circulation), sudorific, tonic, vermifuge.

COMPATIBILITIES
It blends well with bergamot, lemon, rosemary, melissa, lavender, lavandin, marjoram, Peru balsam, and pine.

SAFETY DATA
Contraindicated in cases of high blood pressure. Red thyme oil, serpolet (from wild thyme), "thymol" and "carvacrol" type oils all contain quite large amounts of toxic phenols (carvacrol and thymol). White thyme is not a "complete" oil and is often adulterated. Lemon thyme and "linalol" types are in general less toxic, nonirritant, with less possibility of sensitization – safe for use on the skin and with children

TILIA X VULGARIS

Linden

FAMILY: TILIACEAE

Herbal/Folk Tradition

Linden tea, known as "tilleul", is drunk a great deal in continental Europe, as a general relaxant. The flowers are also used for indigestion, palpitations, nausea, hysteria, and catarrh following a cold. Linden honey is highly regarded.

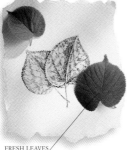

FRESH LEAVES

A tall graceful tree up to 98ft (30m) high with a smooth bark, spreading branches, and bright green, heart-shaped leaves. It has yellowy-white flowers borne in clusters, which have a very powerful scent.

DATAFILE

AROMATHERAPY/ HOME USE
Digestive System: *Cramps, indigestion, liver pains.*
Nervous System: *Headaches, insomnia, migraine, nervous tension, and stress-related conditions.*

EXTRACTION
A concrete and absolute by solvent extraction from the dried flowers.

ACTIONS
Astringent, antispasmodic, bechic, carminative, cephalic, diaphoretic, diuretic, emollient, nervine, sedative, tonic.

Tilia x vulgaris Native to Europe and the northern hemisphere. Common in Britain, France, and the Netherlands.

SAFETY DATA

Most products are adulterated or synthetic. No safety data available at present

TRACHYSPERMUM COPTICUM

Ajowan

FAMILY: APIACEAE (UMBELLIFERAE)

Herbal/Folk Tradition

The seeds are used in curry powders and as a household remedy for intestinal problems. The tincture, essential oil, and "thymol" are used in India for cholera.

AJOWAN SEEDS

An annual herb with a grayish-brown seed. It has bright green leaves and an erect habit of growth usually not exceeding 20in (50cm) in height. It is an umbelliferous plant, widely cultivated in India for medicinal properties.

DATAFILE

AROMATHERAPY/ HOME USE
Not recommended.

EXTRACTION
Essential oil by steam distillation from the seed.

ACTIONS
Powerful antiseptic and germicide, carminative.

SAFETY DATA

Possible mucous membrane and dermal irritant. Due to high thymol level, should be avoided in pregnancy. Toxicity levels are unknown

TSUGA CANADENSIS

Hemlock spruce

FAMILY: PINACEAE

Herbal/Folk Tradition

The bark of the hemlock spruce is current in the *British Herbal Pharmacopoeia* indicated for diarrhea, cystitis, mucous colitis, leucorrhea, uterine prolapse, pharyngitis, stomatitis and gingivitis.

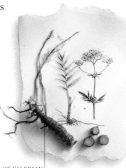

NEWLY FORMED CONES

FRESH HEMLOCK SPRUCE | FRESH LEAVES

A large evergreen tree up to 164ft (50m) tall, with slender horizontal branches, finely toothed leaves, and smallish brown cones. It yields a natural exudation from its bark.

DATAFILE

AROMATHERAPY/ HOME USE
Circulation, Muscles, and Joints: *Muscular aches and pains, poor circulation, rheumatism.*
Respiratory System: *Asthma, bronchitis, coughs, respiratory weakness.*
Immune System: *Colds, flu, infections.*
Nervous System: *Anxiety, stress-related conditions.*

EXTRACTION
Essential oil by steam distillation from the needles and twigs.

ACTIONS
Antimicrobial, antiseptic, antitussive, astringent, diaphoretic, diuretic, expectorant, nervine, rubefacients, tonic.

COMPATIBILITIES
It blends well with pine, oakmoss, cedarwood, galbanum, benzoin, lavender, lavandin, and rosemary.

SAFETY DATA
Nontoxic, nonirritant, nonsensitizing

VALERIANA FAURIEI

Valerian

FAMILY: VALERIANACEAE

Herbal/Folk Tradition

This herb, highly esteemed since medieval times, has been used in the West for complaints where there is nervous tension, such as insomnia, and migraine, and as a pain reliever.

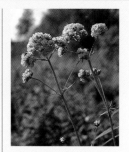

Valeriana fauriei

ROOT OF VALERIAN

A perennial herb up to 5ft (1.5m) high with a hollow, erect stem, deeply dissected dark leaves, and many purplish-white flowers. It has short, thick, grayish roots, largely showing above ground, which have a strong odor.

DATAFILE

AROMATHERAPY/ HOME USE
Nervous System: *Insomnia, nervous indigestion, migraine, restlessness, and tension states.*

EXTRACTION
Essential oil by steam distillation from the rhizomes. An absolute and concrete by solvent extraction of rhizomes.

ACTIONS
Anodyne, antidandruff, diuretic, antispasmodic, bactericidal, carminative, depressant of the central nervous system, hypnotic, hypotensive, regulator, sedative, stomachic.

COMPATIBILITIES
It blends well with patchouli, costus, oakmoss, pine, lavender, cedarwood, mandarin, petitgrain, and rosemary.

SAFETY DATA
Nontoxic, nonirritant, possible sensitization. Use in moderation

Vanilla

FAMILY: ORCHIDACEAE

Herbal/Folk Tradition

When vanilla is grown in cultivation, the deep trumpet-shaped flowers have to be hand-pollinated – except in Mexico where the native humming birds do most of the work!

DRIED VANILLA BEAN

A perennial herbaceous climbing vine up to 82ft (25m) high, with green stems and large white flowers that have a deep narrow trumpet. The green capsules or fruits are picked and "cured". The immature vanilla "pod" or "bean" is fermented and dried to turn it into a fragrant brown vanilla bean.

DATAFILE

AROMATHERAPY/ HOME USE
None.

EXTRACTION
A resinoid (often called an oleoresin) by solvent extraction from the "cured" vanilla beans. (An absolute is occasionally produced by further extraction from the resinoid.)

ACTIONS
Balsamic.

COMPATIBILITIES
It blends well with sandalwood, vetiver, opopanax, benzoin, balsams, and spice oils.

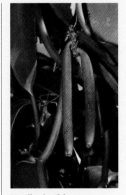

*Vanilla planifolia
Native to Central America and Mexico.*

SAFETY DATA
Nontoxic, common sensitizing agent. Widely adulterated

Vetiver

FAMILY: POACEAE (GRAMINEAE)

Herbal/Folk Tradition

The rootlets have been used in the East for their fine fragrance since antiquity. They are used by the locals to protect domestic animals from vermin. In India and Sri Lanka the essence is known as "the oil of tranquillity".

FRESH VETIVER GRASS

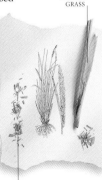

DRIED VETIVER GRASS

A tall, tufted, perennial, scented grass, with a straight stem, long, narrow leaves, and an abundant, complex lacework of underground white rootlets.

DATAFILE

AROMATHERAPY/ HOME USE
Skin Care: *Acne, cuts, oily skin, wounds.*
Circulation, Muscles, and Joints: *Arthritis, muscular aches and pains, rheumatism, sprains, stiffness.*
Nervous System: *Debility, depression, insomnia, nervous tension – Vetiver is deeply relaxing, and is a valuable oil in massage and baths for anybody suffering from stress.*

EXTRACTION
Essential oil by steam distillation from the roots and rootlets – washed, chopped, dried, and soaked. A resinoid is produced by solvent extraction for perfumery work.

ACTIONS
Antiseptic, antispasmodic, depurative, rubefacient, sedative (nervous system), stimulant (circulatory, production of red corpuscles), tonic, vermifuge.

COMPATIBILITIES
It blends well with sandalwood, rose, violet, jasmine, opopanax, patchouli, oakmoss, lavender, clary sage, mimosa, cassie, and ylang ylang.

SAFETY DATA
Nontoxic, nonirritant, nonsensitizing

VIOLA ODORATA
Violet
FAMILY: VIOLACEAE

Herbal/Folk Tradition
Both the leaf and flowers have a long tradition of use in herbal medicine, mainly for congestive pulmonary conditions and sensitive skin conditions. The leaf has also been used to treat cystitis and as a mouthwash for infections of the mouth and throat.

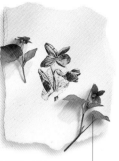

FLOWERING SPRIG OF VIOLET

A small, tender, perennial plant with dark green, heart-shaped leaves, fragrant violet-blue flowers, and an oblique underground rhizome.

DATAFILE	
AROMATHERAPY/ HOME USE	**EXTRACTION**
Skin Care: *Acne, eczema, refiines the pores, thread veins, wounds.*	A concrete and absolute from fresh leaves or flowers.
Circulation, Muscles, and Joints: *Fibrosis, poor circulation, rheumatism.*	**ACTIONS**
Respiratory System: *Bronchitis, catarrh, mouth and throat infections.*	Analgestic (mild), anti-inflammatory, antirheumatic, antiseptic, decongestant (liver), diuretic, expectorant, laxative, soporific, stimulant (circulation).
Nervous System: *Dizziness, headaches, insomnia, nervous exhaustion – the scent was believed to comfort and strengthen the heart.*	**COMPATIBILITIES** It blends well with tuberose, clary sage, boronia, tarragon, cumin, hop, basil, hyacinth, and other florals.

SAFETY DATA
Nontoxic, nonirritant, possible sensitization in some individuals

ZINGIBER OFFICINALE
Ginger
FAMILY: ZINGIBERACEAE

Herbal/Folk Tradition
Ginger has been used as a spice and as a remedy for thousands of years. In China fresh ginger is used for complaints ranging from to malaria to rheumatism. It is best known as a digestive aid.

GROUND GINGER

SECTION OF ROOT

RHIZOME ROOT

An erect perennial herb up to 3ft (1m) high with a thick, spreading, pungent tuberous rhizome. Each year it sends up a green reedlike stalk with narrow spear-shaped leaves and white or yellow flowers on a spike direct from the root.

DATAFILE	
AROMATHERAPY/ HOME USE	**EXTRACTION**
Circulation, Muscles, and Joints: *Arthritis, fatigue, muscular aches and pains, poor circulation, rheumatism, sprains, strains, etc.*	Essential oil by steam distillation from unpeeled, dried ground, root.
Respiratory System: *Catarrh, congestion, coughs, sinusitis, sore throat.*	**ACTIONS** Analgesic, antioxidant, antiseptic, antispasmodic, antitussive, aperitif,
Digestive System: *Diarrhea, colic, cramp, flatulence, indigestion, loss of appetite, nausea, travel sickness.*	aphrodisiac, bactericidal, carminative, cephalic, diaphoretic, expectorant, febrifuge, laxative, rubefacient, stimulant, stomachic.
Immune System: *Chills, colds, flu, fever, infectious disease.*	**COMPATIBILITIES**
Nervous System: *Debility, nervous exhaustion.*	It blends well with sandalwood, vetiver, patchouli, frankincense, rosewood, cedarwood, coriander, rose, lime, orange blossom, orange, and other citrus oils.

SAFETY DATA
Nontoxic, nonirritant (except in high concentration), slightly phototoxic; may cause sensitization in some individuals

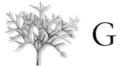

Glossary

Abortifacient: capable of inducing abortion.

Absolute: a highly concentrated viscous, semisolid, or solid perfume material, usually obtained by alcohol extraction from the concrete.

Allergy: hypersensitivity caused by a foreign substance.

Alterative: corrects disordered bodily function.

Amenorrhea: absence of menstruation.

Analgesic: remedy that deadens pain.

Anemia: deficiency in either quality or quantity of red corpuscles in the blood.

Annual: refers to a plant that completes its life cycle in one year.

Anodyne: stills pain and quiets disturbed feelings.

Anthelmintic: a vermifuge, destroying or expelling intestinal worms.

Antibiotic: prevents the growth of, or destroys, bacteria.

Antiemetic: an agent that reduces the incidence and severity of nausea.

Antihemorrhagic: an agent that prevents or combats hemorrhage or bleeding.

Antihistamine: treats allergic conditions; counteracts effects of histamine (produces capillary dilation).

Antimicrobial: an agent that resists or destroys pathogenic microorganisms.

Antioxidant: a substance used to prevent or delay oxidation or deterioration, especially with exposure to air.

Antiphlogistic: checks or counteracts inflammation.

Antipruritic: relieves sensation of itching or prevents its occurrence.

Antipyretic: reduces fever.

Antisclerotic: helps prevent the hardening of tissue.

Antiseborrheic: helps control the products of sebum, the oily secretion from sweat glands.

Antitoxic: an antidote or treatment that counteracts the effects of poison.

Antitussive: relieves coughs.

Aperient: a mild laxative.

Aphonia: loss of voice.

Apoplexy: sudden loss of consciousness, a stroke, or sudden, severe hemorrhage.

Aril: the husk or membrane covering the seed of a plant.

Aromatherapy: the therapeutic use of essential oils.

Arteriosclerosis: loss of elasticity in the artery walls due to thickening.

Astringent: causes contraction of organic tissues.

Atony: lessening or lack of muscle tone.

Axil: upper angle between a stem and leaf or bract.

Bactericidal: an agent that destroys bacteria.

Balsam: a resinous semisolid mass or viscous liquid exuded from a plant. A "true" balsam has a high content of benzoic acid, benzoates, cinnamic acid, or cinnamates.

Balsamic: a soothing medicine or application.

Bechic: anything that relieves or cures coughs; or referring to cough.

Biennial: a plant that completes its life cycle in two years, without flowering in the first year.

Bilious: a condition caused by an excessive secretion of bile.

Calmative: a sedative.

Calyx: the sepals or outer layer of floral leaves.

Capsule: a dry fruit, opening when ripe, composed of more than one carpel.

Cardiac: pertaining to the heart.

Carminative: settles the digestive system, relieves flatulence.

Chemotype: the same botanical species occurring in other forms due to different conditions of growth

Cholagogue: stimulates the secretion and flow of bile into the duodenum.

Cholecystokinetic: agent that stimulates the contraction of the gall bladder.

Choleretic: aids excretion of bile by the liver, so there is a greater flow of bile.

Cholesterol: a steroid alcohol found in nervous tissue, red blood cells, animal fat, and bile.

Cicatrizant: an agent that promotes healing by the formation of scar tissue.

Cirrhosis: degeneration in any organ (especially liver), caused by various poisons, bacteria, or other agents, resulting in fibrous tissue overgrowth.

Colic: pain due to contraction of the muscle of the abdominal organs.

Colitis: inflammation of the colon.

Concrete: a concentrate, waxy, solid, or semisolid perfume material made from previously live plant matter, usually using a hydrocarbon type of solvent.

Corolla: the petals of a flower.

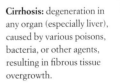

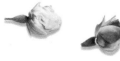

Cutaneous: pertaining to the skin.

Cystitis: bladder inflammation, usually characterized by pain on urinating.

Cytophylactic: the process of increasing the activity of leucocytes in defense of the body against infection.

Cytotoxic: toxic to all cells.

Decoction: a herbal preparation, where the plant material is boiled in water and reduced to make a concentration.

Demulcent: a substance that protects mucous membranes and allays irritation.

Depurative: helps combat impurity in the blood and organs; detoxifying.

Dermatitis: inflammation of the skin.

Diuretic: aids production of urine.

Drupe: a fleshy fruit, with one or more seeds, each surrounded by a stony layer.

Dysmenorrhea: painful menstruation.

Edema: a painless swelling caused by fluid retention beneath the skin.

Emetic: induces vomiting.

Emmenagogue: induces or assists menstruation.

Emollient: softens and soothes the skin.

Engorgement: congestion of a part of the tissues, or fullness (as in the breasts).

Enteritis: inflammation of the mucous membrane of the intestine.

Enzyme: complex proteins that are produced by the living cells, and catalyze specific biochemical reactions.

Essential oil: a volatile and aromatic liquid (sometimes semisolid), which generally constitutes the odorous principles of a plant. It is obtained by a process of expression or distillation from a single botanical form or species.

Febrifuge: combats fever.

Fixative: a material that slows down the rate of evaporation of the more volatile components in a perfume composition.

Fixed oil: vegetable oils obtained from plants that are fatty, dense, and non-volatile, such as olive oil.

Follicle: a dry, one-celled, fruit.

Galactagogue: increases milk secretion.

Germicidal: destroys germs or micro-organisms such as bacteria, etc.

Gums: The term "gum" is often applied to "resins." Strictly speaking, gums are natural or synthetic water-soluble materials, such as gum arabic.

Heartwood: central part of a tree trunk.

Hematuria: blood in the urine.

Hemorrhoids: piles, dilated rectal veins.

Hemostatic: arrests bleeding.

Hepatic: relating to the liver.

Herpes: inflammation of the skin or mucous membrane.

Hormone: a product of living cells that produces a specific effect on the activity of cells remote from its point of origin.

Hybrid: a plant created by fertilization of one species or subspecies by another.

Hypertension: raised blood pressure.

Hypocholesterolemia: lowering the cholesterol content of the blood.

Hypoglycemia: lowered blood sugar levels or concentration.

Hypotension: low blood pressure, or a fall in blood pressure.

Inflorescence: flowering structure above the last stem leaves.

Infusion: a herbal remedy prepared by steeping the plant material in water.

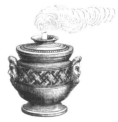

Lanceolate: lance-shaped, oval, and pointed at both ends.

Legume: a fruit consisting of one carpel, opening on one side, such as a pea.

Leucocyte: white blood cells responsible for fighting disease.

Leucocytosis: an increase in the number of white blood cells above normal limits.

Leucorrhea: white vaginal discharge.

Ligulet: a narrow protection from the top of a leaf sheath in grasses.

Lipolytic: causing lipolysis, the chemical disintegration or splitting of fats.

Macerate: soak until soft.

Menopause: the normal cessation of menstruation, a life change for women.

Menorrhagia: excessive menstruation.

Metrorrhagia: uterine bleeding outside the menstrual cycle.

Microbe: a minute living organism – pathogenic bacteria, viruses, etc.

Mucilage: a substance containing demulcent gelatinous constituents.

Mucolytic: breaking down mucus.

Narcotic: a substance that induces sleep; intoxicating or poisonous in large doses.

Nervine: strengthening and toning to the nerves and nervous system.

Nephritis: inflammation of the kidneys.

Neuralgia: a stabbing pain along a nerve pathway.

Neurasthenia: nervous exhaustion.

Oleo gum resin: a natural exudation from trees and plants that consists mainly of essential oil, gum, and resin.

Oleoresin: a natural resinous exudation from plants, or an aromatic liquid preparation, extracted from botanical matter using solvents.

Ovate: egg-shaped.

Palpitation: undue awareness of the heartbeat, occasioned by anxiety. Rapid heartbeats or abnormal rhythm.

Pappus: the calyx in a composite flower having feathery hairs, scales, or bristles.

Parturient: aiding childbirth.

Pathogenic: causing or producing disease.

Peptic: applied to gastric secretions and areas affected by them.

Perennial: a plant that lives for more than two years.

Petiole: the stalk of a leaf.

Pharmacology: medical science of drugs.

Pharmacopoeia: an official publication of drugs in common use.

Phytohormones: plant substances that mimic the action of human hormones.

Phytotherapy: the treatment of disease by plants; herbal medicine.

Pinnate: a leaf composed of more than three leaflets arranged in two rows along a common stalk.

Prophylactic: preventative of disease or infection.

Prostatitis: any inflammatory condition of the prostate gland.

Pruritis: itching.

Psoriasis: a skin disease characterized by red patches and silver scaling.

Psychosomatic: the manifestation of physical symptoms resulting from a mental state.

Pulmonary: pertaining to the lungs.

Pyelitis: inflammation of the kidney.

Receptacle: the upper part of the stem from which the floral parts arise.

Rectification: the process of redistillation applied to essential oils to rid them of certain constituents.

Regulator: an agent that helps balance and regulate the functions of the body.

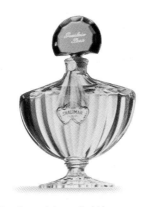

Renal: pertaining to the kidney.

Resins: a natural or prepared product, either solid or semisolid in nature. Natural resins are exudations from trees, such as mastic; prepared resins are oleoresins from which essential oil has been removed.

Resinoids: a perfumery material prepared from natural resinous matter, such as balsams, by extraction with a hydrocarbon type of solvent.

Resolvent: an agent that disperses swelling, or effects absorption of a new growth.

Rhizome: an underground stem lasting more than one season.

Rosette: leaves that are closely arranged in a spiral.

Rubefacient: a substance that causes redness of the skin, possibly irritation.

Sciatica: pain down the back of the legs, in the area supplied by the sciatic nerve.

Sclerosis: hardening of tissue due to inflammation.

Seborrhea: increased secretion of sebum, usually associated with excessive oil secretion from the sweat glands.

Sessile: without a stalk.

Sialogogue: an agent that stimulates the secretion of saliva.

Spike: an inflorescence in which the sessile flowers are arranged in a raceme.

Splenic: relating to the spleen, the largest endocrine gland.

Styptic: an astringent agent that stops or reduces external bleeding.

Sudorific: an agent that causes sweating.

Synergy: agents working together harmoniously.

Tachycardia: abnormally increased heartbeat and pulse rate.

Tannin: an astringent substance that helps seal the tissue.

Thrombosis: formation of a thrombus or blood clot.

Thrush: an infection of the mouth or vaginal region caused by a fungus.

Tincture: a herbal remedy or perfumery material prepared in an alcohol base.

Tracheitis: inflammation of the windpipe.

Trifoliate: a plant having three distinct leaflets.

Tuber: a swollen part of an underground stem of one year's duration, capable of new growth.

Umbel: umbrellalike; a flower where the petioles arise from the stem top

Vermifuge: expels intestinal worms.

Volatile: unstable, evaporates easily, as in "volatile oil"; *see* Essential oil.

Vulnerary: an agent that helps heal wounds and sores by external application.

Whorl: a circle of leaves around a node.

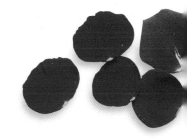

Further Reading

ARCTANDER, S. *Perfume and Flavor Materials of Natural Origin,* published by the author, Elizabeth, New Jersey, 1960.

DE BAIRACLI, LEVY, J. *The Illustrated Herbal Handbook,* Faber & Faber, 1982.

BAERHEIM, S.A. & SCHEFFER, J.J.C. *Essential Oils and Aromatic Plants,* Dr. W. Junk Publications, 1989.

BECKETT, S. *Herbs to Soothe Your Nerves,* Thorsons, 1977.

BERESFORD-COOKE, C. *Massage for Healing and Relaxation,* Arlington, 1986.

BIANCHINI, F. & CORBETTA, F. *Health Plants of the World – Atlas of Medicinal Plants,* Newsweek Books, New York, 1977.

BUCHMAN, D.D. *Feed Your Face,* Duckworth, 1980.

BUCHMAN, D.D. *Herbal Medicine,* Rider, 1984.

CHETWYND, T. *A Dictionary of Symbols,* Paladin, 1982.

CHIEJ, R. *The Macdonald Encyclopedia of Medicinal Plants,* Arnoldo Mondadori, Editore, Milan, 1984.

CONWAY, D. *The Magic of Herbs,* Mayflower, 1973.

COON, N. *The Dictionary of Useful Plants,* Rodale, Emmaus, Pa.,1974.

CULPEPER, N. *Culpeper's Complete Herbal,* W. Foulsham & Co. Ltd, 1952.

DAVIS, P. *Aromatherapy, An A–Z,* C.W. Daniel, 1988.

FAY, I. *Perfumery with Herbs,* Darton, Longman and Todd, 1979.

DOUGLAS, J.S. *Making Your Own Cosmetics,* Pelham Books, 1979.

DOWNING, G. *The Massage Book,* Penguin, 1974.

GRIEVE, M. *A Modern Herbal,* Penguin, 1982.

GRIGGS, B. *The Home Herbal,* Pan, 1983.

GUENTHER, E. *The Essential Oils,* Van Nostrand, New York, 1948.

HALL, R., KLEMME D. & NIENHAUS J. *The H & R Book: Guide to Fragrance Ingredients,* Johnson Publishing, 1985.

HEPPER, C. *Herbal Cosmetics,* Thorsons, 1987.

HERITEATU, J. *Potpourris and other Fragrant Delights,* Penguin, 1975.

HOFFMAN, D. *The New Holistic Herbal,* Element Books, 1990.

HUXLEY, A. *Natural Beauty With Herbs,* Darton, Longman and Todd, 1977.

JESSEE, J.E. *Perfume Album,* Robert E. Krieger, 1974.

LAUTIE, R. & PASSEBECQ, A. *Aromatherapy; the Use of Plant Essences in Healing,* Thorsons, 1982.

LAVABRE, M. *Aromatherapy Workbook,* Healing Arts Press, Vermont, 1990.

LAWRENCE, B.M. *Essential Oils,* Allured Publishing Co., Wheaton, USA, 1978.

LEUNG, A.Y. *Encyclopedia of Common Natural Ingredients,* John Wiley, New York, 1980.

LITTLE, K. *Kitty Little's Book of Herbal Beauty,* Penguin, 1980.

MAURY, M. *Marguerite Maury's Guide to Aromatherapy,* C.W. Daniel, 1989.

MABEY, R. *The Complete New Herbal,* Elm Tree Books, 1988.

METCALFE, J. *Herbs and Aromatherapy,* Webb & Bower, 1989.

MILLS, S.Y. *The A–Z of Modern Herbalism,* Thorsons, 1989.

NAVES, Y.R. & MAZUYER, G. *Natural Perfume Materials,* Reinhold Publishing, New York, 1947.

PAGE, M. *The Observers Book of Herbs,* Frederick Warne, 1980.

PRICE, S. *Practical Aromatherapy,* Thorsons, 1983.

ROSE, F. *The Wild Flower Key,* Frederick Warne, 1981.

RYMAN, D. *The Aromatherapy Handbook,* Century, 1984.

STEAD, C. *The Power of Holistic Aromatherapy,* Javelin Books, 1986.

STOBART, T. *Herbs, Spices and Flavourings,* Penguin, 1979.

LE STRANGE, R. *A History of Herbal Plants,* Angus and Robertson, 1977.

THOMSON, W.A.R. *Healing Plants – A Modern Herbal,* Macmillan, 1978.

TISSERAND, R. *The Essential Oil Safety Data Manual,* The Association of Tisserand Aromatherapists, 1985.

TISSERAND, R. *The Art of Aromatherapy,* C.W. Daniel, 1985.

VALNET, J. *The Practice of Aromatherapy,* C.W. Daniel (English Translation), 1982.

WEISS, R.F. *Herbal Medicine,* Arcanum, 1988.

WHITMONT, E.C. *Psyche and Substance,* North Atlantic Books, 1980.

WILLIAMS, D. *Lecture Notes on Essential Oils,* Eve Taylor Ltd, 1989.

WORWOOD, V.A. *The Fragrant Pharmacy,* Macmillan, 1990.

WREN, R.C. *Potters New Cyclopaedia of Botanical Drugs and Preparations,* C.W. Daniel, 1988.

References

1. BAERHEIM & SCHEFFER. *Essential Oils and Aromatic Plants.*

2. TISSERAND, R. *The Essential Oil Safety Manual*, p.79.

3. LAVABRE, M. *Aromatherapy Workbook*, p.86.

4. DAVIS, P. *Aromatherapy, An A–Z*, p.135.

5. MONCRIEFF, R.W. *Odours*, 1970.

6. MAURY, M. *Marguerite Maury's Guide to Aromatherapy*, p.104.

7. LEUNG, A.Y. *Encyclopedia of Common Natural Ingredients*, p.155.

8. TISSERAND, as above, p.96.

9. DAVIS, as above, p.236.

10. TISSERAND, as above, p.189.

11. GRIEVE, M. *A Modern Herbal*, p.127.

12. LEUNG, A.Y. *Encyclopedia of Common Natural Ingredients*, p.166.

13. GRIEVE, as above.

14. MAURY, as above, p.104.

15. TISSERAND, as above, p.84.

16. CULPEPER, N. *Culpeper's Complete Herbal*, p.202.

17. TISSERAND, R. *The Art of Aromatherapy*, p.238.

18. ARCTANDER, S. *Perfume and Flavor Materials of Natural Origin*, p.581.

19. CULPEPER, as above, p.211.

20. DAVIS, as above, p.328.

21. SCHOOL OF HERBAL MEDICINE, *Materia Medica, Part II*, p.25.

22. HOFFMANN, D. *The New Holistic Herbal*, p.168.

23. CULPEPER, as above, p.298.

24. *British Herbal Pharmacopoeia 1983*, p.181.

25. ARCTANDER, as above, p.563.

26. LEUNG, as above, p.62.

27. ARCTANDER, as above, p.607.

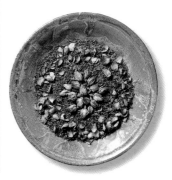

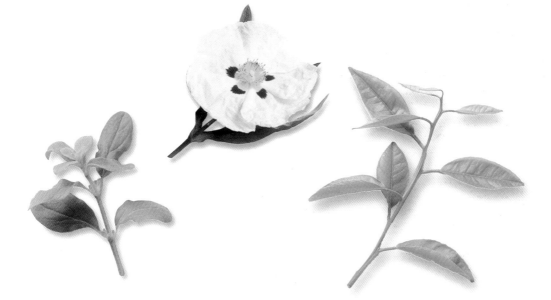

Useful Addresses

A wide selection of top-quality essential oils, base oils, aromatherapy books, and other aromatic products is available from Aqua Oleum UK. International mail order professional and export lists are also offered. Safety information, quality control, and up-to-date product data are outlined in *The Essential Oil Catalogue* supplied free with price list.

Aqua Oleum
Unit 3, Lower Wharf, Wallbridge, Stroud, Glos GL5 3JA, UK
Tel (01453) 753555
Fax (01453) 752179 .

Aqua Oleum products are also available from:

CANADA & USA
Nature Trading Limited
Box 263, 1857 West 4th Avenue, Vancouver, B.C., Canada, V63 1M4

DENMARK & SWEDEN
Urtekram A/S, Klostermarken 20, DK-9550 Mariager, Denmark

FINLAND
Luonnonruokatukku
Aduki Ky, Kirvesmelhankatu 10, 00810 Helsinki, Finland

IRELAND
Wholefoods Wholesale
Unit 2D, Kylemore Industrial Estate, Dublin 10, Republic of Ireland

Soap Opera Ltd
Unit 3, Enterprise Centre, Stafford Street, Nenagh, Co. Tipperary, Republic of Ireland

JAPAN
Marunake K.K.
1-12-4 Ginza Chuo-ku, Tokyo, Japan

HONG KONG
7 Old Bailey Street, Central, Hong Kong

Information regarding qualified aromatherapists and training programmes can be obtained from:

UK
The International Federation of Aromatherapists
Stamford House, 2/4 Chiswick High Road, London, W4 1TH, UK
Tel: 020 8742 2605

USA
The American Alliance of Aromatherapy
PO Box 750428, Petaluma, CA 94975, USA
Tel: (707) 778 6762

AUSTRALIA
The International Federation of Aromatherapists
1/390 Burwood Road, Hawthorne, Melbourne, Victoria 3122, Australia
Tel: (613) 819 2502
Fax: (613) 819 2399

Information regarding qualified medical herbalists and training programs can be obtained from:

UK
The School of Herbal Medicine/Phytotherapy
Bucksteep Manor, Bodle Street Green, Hailsham, Sussex, BN27 4RJ, UK
Tel: (01323) 833 812/4

The National Institute of Medical Herbalists
56 Longbrook Street, Exeter, Devon, EX4 6AH, UK
Tel: (01392) 426022

USA
American Botanical Council and Herb Research Foundation, PO Box 201660, Austin, Texas 78720, USA

California School of Herbal Studies
9309 HWY 116, Forestville, CA 95436, USA

AUSTRALIA
National Herbalists Association of Australia, Suite 305, 3 Smail Street, Broadway, New South Wales 2007, Australia
Tel: (02) 211 6437
Fax: (02) 211 6452

General information on holistic forms of treatment can be obtained from:

UK
British Holistic Medical Association
Trust House, Royal Shrewsbury Hospital South, Shrewsbury, Shropshire, SY3 8XF, UK
Tel: (01743) 261155
Fax: (01743) 353637

USA
American Holistic Medical Association
Suite 201, 4101 Lake Boone Trail, Raleigh, North Carolina 27607, USA
Tel: (919) 787 5146
Fax: (919) 787 4916

CANADA
Canadian Holistic Medical Association
700 Bay Street, PO Box 101, Suite 604, Toronto, Ontario , M5G 1Z6, Canada

AUSTRALIA
Australian Natural Therapists Association, PO Box 308, Melrose Park, South Australia 5039
Tel: 8297 9533
Fax: 8297 0003

Index

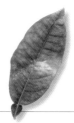